T0312611

MEDICINE MANAGEMENT SKILLS
FOR NURSES

Student Survival Skills Series

Survive your nursing course with these essential guides for all student nurses:

Calculation Skills for Nurses
Claire Boyd
9781118448892

Medicine Management Skills for Nurses
Claire Boyd
9781118448854

Clinical Skills for Nurses
Claire Boyd
9781118448779

MEDICINE MANAGEMENT SKILLS
FOR NURSES

Second Edition

Claire Boyd
RGN, Cert Ed
Practice Development Trainer

WILEY Blackwell

Registered Offices
John Wiley & Sons, Inc., 111 River Street, Hoboken, NJ 07030, USA
John Wiley & Sons Ltd, The Atrium, Southern Gate, Chichester, West Sussex, PO19 8SQ, UK

Editorial Office
9600 Garsington Road, Oxford, OX4 2DQ, UK

For details of our global editorial offices, customer services, and more information about Wiley products visit us at www.wiley.com.

Wiley also publishes its books in a variety of electronic formats and by print-on-demand. Some content that appears in standard print versions of this book may not be available in other formats.

Library of Congress Cataloging-in-Publication Data applied for

PB ISBN: 9781119807926

Cover Design: Wiley
Cover Images: © chuwy/Getty Images, © rambo182/Getty Images

Set in 9/12pt Trade Gothic Light by Straive, Pondicherry, India

Printed and bound in Great Britain by Bell and Bain Ltd, Glasgow

10 9 8 7 6 5 4 3 2 1

Contents

CONTENTS

Preface

This book is designed to assist the student healthcare worker in the field of medicines management. All exercises are related to practice and the healthcare environment. It is full of medicines management information you will need as a healthcare professional.

The book looks at the general principles of drug administration, and features 'how to' chapters covering the administration of many types of drug. All the material has been requested by students like you, who told me what they wanted in a medicines management book. It is designed to be a quick reference, one on which you can build your knowledge and skills.

At the start of your nursing career you will observe drug administration and then gradually take a more active part in the process. Don't shy away from this, as one day you will be on your own and the patient will rely on you as being the fount of all knowledge.

Nobody expects you to be all knowing at the start of your career and you will need to have quite a few drug-related competencies signed off to prove your ability during your training. Many clinical areas also supply students with an induction pack during placement. This pack usually has a section on commonly prescribed medications used in that area. It is from this that you will build up your knowledge of cardiac drugs, renal drugs, drugs used in neurosurgical wards, drugs used in paediatric care, and so on.

The book talks about patients but often uses the community terminology of service user as well. The paediatric nurse has not been forgotten, with information throughout incorporating this branch of nursing.

PREFACE

The book incorporates many exercises to check understanding, to help you to build confidence and competence. It has been also compiled using quotes and tips from student nurses themselves: a book by students for students.

Claire Boyd
Bristol

Introduction

Hello all, my name is Claire and I have been a nurse and Practice Development Trainer in a large Nation Health Service (NHS) trust for over 30 years (I started very young)! This is the second edition of this book which is jam-packed with information – filled to the rafters with information in a book small enough to be carried around and referred to without weighing a ton and giving you a hernia!

Chatting to nursing staff, just like you, I have often been told that they have real fears about all aspects of medicines management. These fears are especially with regard to the administration of drugs, knowing that this is a skill they will have to acquire and use throughout their chosen career. Does this sound like you? Are you a little over-awed with the prospect of being let loose in your clinical area to administer drugs to the patients?

To add to the fear factor, many students complain that they are often unable to practice their drug-administration competences under supervision due to the ever-increasing demands on the preceptor (wait until you become one and see how hard it is!). They tell me that they are not getting adequate input in the area of medicines management during their training, so their thinking is, 'how am I meant to get my competences signed off, let alone become confident and competent?'

No need to fear: this book will at least give you the knowledge behind the skill, increasing your confidence and competence prior to really getting stuck in with the 'hands-on' element in your clinical area. In short, this book is designed to support you, the **Student Nurse** as well as those who are newly qualified – the **Newly Qualified Nurse** (NQN) – congratulations on your wonderful achievement. Also, with the ever-changing face of health care, it is also aimed at those of you who are now expected to administer medications, namely the **Assistant Practitioners** and to the newer members of our family the **Nursing Associate** and the **Non-Medical Nurse Prescriber** (NMP). This book is also for those of you coming back into nursing – The **Return to Practice Nurse** and **Overseas Nurses** – welcome all!

This book contains the information and exercises I deliver to healthcare professionals during their medicines management training. I hope that I have made the writing style informal but brief, as though I am sitting beside you to help you along the way. All the answers to the activities, questions, and 'Test your Knowledge' exercises can be found at the back of the book.

Remembering my own time as a student nurse, it was being let loose with the drug trolley that most scared me: what if I made a mistake? Times have not changed, as many of you have informed me that you need a book to increase your theoretical knowledge, as well as to advise on the practicalities.

Throughout the book students have added their own words of wisdom, in the form of tips for their peers from their own experiences, or queries they may have had. I have also taken on board subjects you wanted added to this second edition:

- Web resources added to chapters – tick
- Oxygen therapy information added – tick
- More case studies – tick
- Drugs that may contribute to falls in frail adults – tick
- More on cultural considerations in medicines management – tick

The book is designed to take you from your first day 'on the job' to your qualification, and beyond. It covers all areas of medicines management, for the acute hospital to the community, adults, and paediatrics.

Nursing is a dynamic field and the book is evidence-based and looks at the theory and practice of drug administration briefly and coherently. The pharmaceutical industry is forever evolving and new drugs are coming onto the market regularly. Take time to talk to your patients to gain an understanding of drugs you may not have seen before. Pick up the new editions of the *British National Formulary* or go on-line to access it (adult and paediatric editions) and dip into this source of information regularly.

Please remember that there are many areas within the clinical skill of drug administration that a student is not permitted to undertake. For instance, you may not give intravenous drugs. This does not mean that you can't observe these drugs being prepared and administered by professionals. Never perform any task that you are not permitted to undertake, even if you are asked to do so.

My final tip to you is never administer a drug to anyone without knowing what it does and why it has been prescribed and all the contra indications. Lastly, take your time when administering medicines and never cut corners.

Acknowledgements

As always, first acknowledgements go to the healthcare workers (Nurses, Nursing Associates, Assistant Practitioners, etc). I have had the honour of teaching in the skill of medicines management. As with the other books in the Series, it is their tips and quotes that have been used throughout the book. In short, what you wanted in a Medicines Management book.

Thanks also go to Magenta Styles (Executive Editor at Wiley Blackwell) for her guidance, and to the team at Wiley's for all their assistance and support.

This book is dedicated to my loving family: my wonderful husband Rob (for the photographs), Simon and Louise and David for allowing me to use photographs of their body parts: nose, ears, eyes, and fingers (what did you think I meant?). To my gorgeous grandsons Owen and Rhys – the light of our lives. Thank you, my family, for supporting me in my book-writing foray.

The 24-Hour Clock

Time	24-hour clock
1 a.m.	01:00
2 a.m.	02:00
3 a.m.	03:00
4 a.m.	04:00
5 a.m.	05:00
6 a.m.	06:00
7 a.m.	07:00
8 a.m.	08:00
9 a.m.	09:00
10 a.m.	10:00
11 a.m.	11:00
12 midday	12:00
1 p.m.	13:00
2 p.m.	14:00
3 p.m.	15:00
4 p.m.	16:00
5 p.m.	17:00
6 p.m.	18:00
7 p.m.	19:00
8 p.m.	20:00
9 p.m.	21:00
10 p.m.	22:00
11 p.m.	23:00
12 midnight	24:00

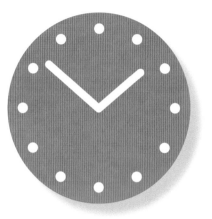

Chapter 1
DRUG ADMINISTRATION: GENERAL PRINCIPLES

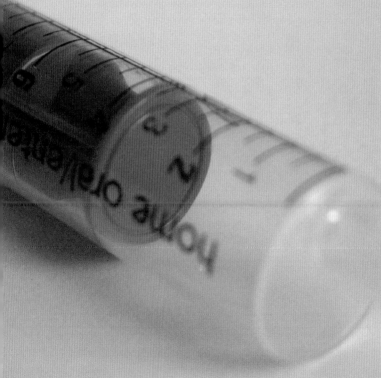

Medicine Management Skills for Nurses, Second Edition. Claire Boyd.
© 2022 John Wiley & Sons Ltd. Published 2022 by John Wiley & Sons Ltd.

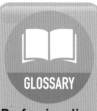

GLOSSARY

Professionalism in nursing

Nurses are expected to display competent and skilful behaviour.

PROFESSIONALISM

You may well worry about making mistakes. Everyone is human after all and prone to error (known as 'Human Factors'). The key is to minimise where the faults can occur. As health carers we *always* put the patient first and apply our professionalism. As with any clinical skill we need to highlight the importance of vigilance, knowledge, and professionalism when administering drugs, as many drug errors occur when staff fail to follow correct procedures or do not recognise the limitations of their own knowledge and skill. Let's look at the cost of drug errors, both monetary and to the individual.

PROFESSIONAL JUDGEMENT

When administering medication, we need to be aware of the following:

- It is not solely a mechanistic task to be performed in strict compliance with the written prescription of a medical practitioner.
- It requires thought and the exercise of professional judgement (Lister, Hofland, and Grafton 2020).

What does this actually mean? Let's look at an example.

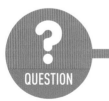

QUESTION

Question 1.1   If a patient has senna and lactulose prescribed and informs you that they have opened their bowels four times that day, do you administer their prescribed laxatives?

Also remember, it is very easy to get distracted, and lose concentration in the clinical area, so always concentrate on the job in hand.

MEDICATION ERRORS

What is a drug error? Well, the Department of Health informs us that:

> A medication error is any *preventable* event that may cause or lead to inappropriate medication use or patient harm while the medication is in the control of health professional, patient, or consumer.

Because nurses predominately administer drugs, they are often the last potential barrier between a medication error and serious harm to a patient, with drug errors frequently featuring in professional misconduct cases.

It is estimated that there are more than 230 million medication errors per year in the National Health Service (NHS). The cost to the NHS was estimated at £98.5 million for the 712 confirmed deaths from drug errors in hospital. However, if we add on the extra cost of patients made seriously ill, or potentially killed by drug errors in primary care, the estimated cost to the NHS is £1.6 billion (yes – billion!) equating to 3.8 million bed days.

So, why do drug errors occur? Well, we have been informed from the same report giving us the facts and figures above that they occur due to:

- Failure to properly monitor patients on powerful drugs,
- Poor communication between general practitioner (GP)'s and hospitals,
- Giving patients the wrong medication.

We also know that mistakes happen due to:

- Drugs that look or sound alike,
- High staff workload,
- Low staffing levels,
- Inexperienced staff.

As a means to combat some of these medication errors, the UK government pledged an investment of £75 million to implement electronic prescribing in hospitals.

Drug Errors and Adverse Reactions

The NHS has graded drug errors and adverse reactions, as follows:

1. Medication errors that do not result in patient harm, i.e. near misses (example: a dose of 500 mg amoxycillin is prepared instead of 250 mg, but corrected before reaching the patient).
2. Medication errors that result in patient harm (example: giving an antibiotic to a patient with a known allergy to that drug).
3. An adverse drug reaction that is not the result of a medication error (example: giving antibiotics to a patient with no previous history of drug reactions, but who then reacts: this is the only non-preventable type of mistake).

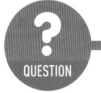

Question 1.2   What is a near miss? Think of an example.

Question 1.3   Apart from killing the patient, what is the worst thing you can do when you have made a drug error?

Worldwide Facts and Figures

Some facts and figures concerning drug errors worldwide:

- Worldwide: 17% of medication errors involve errors in calculations.
- Almost 50% of all intravenous injections feature a mistake, and the number of patients requiring intravenous therapy is increasing.

In medicines management, not only do we have to contend with long, hard to pronounce drug names, but we need to get our heads around all the abbreviations, including Latin ones!

LATIN ABBREVIATIONS

We have all seen the medic on the TV hospital soap opera shouting 'adrenaline stat!' in the emergency room but what does 'stat' actually mean? Well, it means we need to be conversant with Latin abbreviations, that's what it means.

Have a go at seeing how many of the Latin abbreviations you know in Activity 1.1.

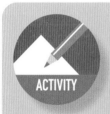

Activity 1.1

Here is a list of Latin abbreviations used when prescribing. What do they mean?

STAT	OM	QDS
AC	ON	QQH
BD	PC	TDS
OD	PRN	TID

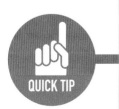

We tend to use specific accepted abbreviations in health care to do with medicines, such as mg, *pro re nata* (PRN), IV, etc. but not mcg as we write microgrammes in full so as not to get confused with mg. Healthcare workers are told not to use abbreviations in their written care plans, medical records, etc. as mistakes can happen. Terms may have two meanings: for instance, DOA can be taken to mean dead on arrival *or* date of admission.

MEDICAL ABBREVIATIONS

There are many medical abbreviations you will see in practice in patients' medical notes. You will also see them used throughout this book. See how many of them you can work out. Don't worry if it is all alien to you, you can find the answers at the back of this book.

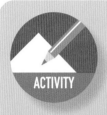

Activity 1.2

AF	DKA	INR
BNF	DM	MAOI
BP	DVT	MHRA
CHD	GI	MI
COPD	GTN	NG
CR	IDDM	NHS
DH	NMC	NICE
NPSA	OTC	NIDDM
NSAID	WHO	PEG
PPI	GP	CD

DID YOU KNOW?

Doctors would often write abbreviations in patients notes – often being very derogatory to them! Thankfully this practice is not seen so much today. Here are just a few:

- LOBNH   Lights on but nobody home
- TEETH   Tried everything else, try homoeopathy
- PIP   Pyjama Induced Paralysis
- TMB   Too many birthdays

DRUG WASTAGE

It has been found that Primary Care Trusts could save almost £7 million each year if GPs prescribed more efficiently. Wastage costs the NHS approximately £200 million. I'm sure we have all met the elderly neighbour with bottles of pills dating back 10 years or more collecting dust in their bathroom cabinets. As health carers we all need to deliver better patient education, explaining why that course of antibiotics that the GP prescribed needs to be completed, even if the patient is feeling better.

Here's a question: what do you think about schemes to recycle drugs back to the pharmacist to be redistributed to other patients? What if the bottles have been opened and the drugs spilled over a dirty floor and put back in the bottle (perhaps even licked by the dog!). Would *you* like to take them? Only use sealed bottles and unopened blister packs, I hear you say, but what if these had been stored on top of a heater for the last six months and their active ingredients have now become unstable?

MEDICATION PROCESS

The medication process is made up of four parts.

*   **Prescribing**: it is often the nurse who notices that a doctor has prescribed something to which the patient is allergic, perhaps because the nurse knows the patient better.
*   **Dispensing and preparation**: a nurse should not use trade names for drugs as confusion may occur, for example Voltarol instead of diclofenac sodium. Perhaps the pharmacist has reconstituted the medication with the wrong transport medium, for example sodium chloride instead of water for injection.
*   **Administration**: you need to be very clear which route a medication should be given through and that the dose has been calculated correctly.
*   **Monitoring**: you need to check the administration and effect of a medicine on the patient. For example, a patient prescribed diclofenac sodium must be checked

to see whether they are asthmatic. Patients with hypertension or heart failure must be monitored carefully if they are given diuretics. Blood pressure, fluid input and output, and sodium and potassium, etc. must be checked.

Any one of these categories could be the weak link where a mistake can occur.

The Department of Health reports that the wrong dose, strength, or frequency of a drug accounts for over a quarter of all medication incident reports.

COMPLEMENTARY MEDICATION

What about complementary medication? As well as a nurse/ nurse educator, I am also a complementary therapist and I am surprised at the number of individuals taking 'natural' remedies and not being aware of their interactions with more mainstream medications: Anticoagulants may react with ginseng, ginkgo Biloba (for improved memory and brain circulation) and should be discontinued 36 hours prior to surgery. Other complementary remedies that need to be considered in the conventional healthcare environment are:

Homoeopathic remedies – individuals may be advised to avoid coffee, peppermint, or menthol as these substances may counteract the effect of the homoeopathic remedy.
St. Johns Wort – which is often used to treat depression, may be harmful for individuals with bipolar disease as it may induce mania.
Liquorice root – should be avoided for those with chronic heart failure and those with hypertension.

Other food/drug interactions can be seen in Chapter 2. Very often complementary therapies are referred to as 'alternative therapy' as they may not be considered part of mainstream healthcare and this is known as CAMS (Complimentary and Alternative Medicine). If in any doubt speak to a pharmacist who can give advice. Never give a drug if you are unsure. Seek advice. Table 1.1 lists many of the complementary therapies which patients may discuss with you. See how many you have heard of:

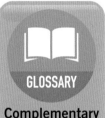

GLOSSARY

Complementary medicine

A broad term used to describe medicines used in *conjunction* with conventional medicine.

Alternative medicine

A broad term used to describe medicines used *instead* of conventional medicine.

Table 1.1 CAMS.

Osteopathy	Chiropractic	Acupuncture
Herbal medicine	Homoeopathy	Aromatherapy
Alexander technique	Massage	Counselling and mindfulness
Iridology	Stress therapy	Hypnotherapy
Reflexology	Shiatsu	Meditation
Relaxation therapy	Thermal auricular therapy	Traditional Chinese and Ayurvedic medicine
Crystal therapy	Colour therapy	Kinesiology

Drug Administration Routes

When administering medications, we also need to be completely conversant with the mode of administration, or route. A very sad case involved a young boy called Wayne Jowett who died as a result of being given his medication intrathecal 'ITH' instead of intravenously (which is written as 'IV').

If you saw the route written as 'ITH' on a prescription chart, what do you think this would mean? Let's look at this and other abbreviations that you may encounter.

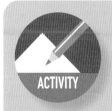

Activity 1.3

Here is a list of abbreviations for routes of drug administration. Can you work out what they mean?

1	ITH	4	IV	7	INH
2	SC	5	IM	8	NEB
3	ID	6	O	9	TOP

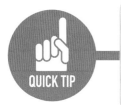

In many NHS Trusts, very few abbreviations are permitted to be used on a drug chart: subcutaneous (SC), intramuscular (IM), IV, O, nebulisation (NEB), topical (TOP), and inhalation (INH). Everything else has to be written out in full so that mistakes don't get made.

Keeping Updated

As well as being conversant with the route abbreviations, if we are administering drugs we need to keep ourselves updated about changes to drug names, as well as contraindications.

Paracetamol (derived from coal tar; also known as acetaminophen) can now be given by the intravenous route, but is obviously much more expensive than oral paracetamol and has a shorter half-life. This means that it is less effective over a longer time span and, as pain is considered to be the fifth vital sign, we need to be aware of this when keeping our patients comfortable and pain free.

Single-Nurse Administration

In most adult hospital settings, it is one nurse who administers the medications to the patients. This is considered to be the safest option as it thought that the lone nurse will take extra care due to their sole responsibility. The exception to this is often injected drugs and controlled drugs, whereby two nurses check and sign for the drug and go to the patient's bedside together to administer the drug.

When there are any calculations or working out to do, two nurses should also check their workings out to agree on the correct answer and dose that the patient requires.

PAEDIATRIC PATIENTS

When medication errors occur, paediatric patients have a higher risk of death than adults due to the fact that most drugs are developed in concentrations for adults,

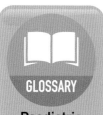

necessitating often complex weight-based calculations for paediatric doses and dilutions. Many drugs are not licensed for use in children. The gastric pH of children only reaches the same level as that of adults when they reach two to three years of age. The British National Formulary (BNF) classifies children into four groups:

- Neonates (up to one month)
- Infants (up to one year)
- One to six years of age
- 6–12 years of age

One of the special safeguards the paediatric clinical areas often have in place is that two nurses have to check and sign the prescription chart. One of these should be a Registered Paediatric Nurse.

GLOSSARY

Paediatric patients

These patients are infants, children, and adolescents.

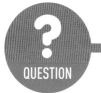

QUESTION

Question 1.4   Other than paediatric patients, who may be considered as another high-risk group?

Older Adults

Ageing can influence many aspects of absorption, distribution, metabolism, and excretion (ADME) with excretion the most affected. This is because by the age of 65, the human kidney is almost a third less efficient than younger adults. This can lead to drugs not being cleared as efficiently from the kidneys, building up, and causing toxicity. Another cause for concern is the effects and side-effects of some drugs which may contribute to falls in frail adults due to postural hypotension and other factors.

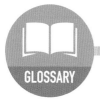

GLOSSARY

Postural hypotension

A form of low blood pressure that happens when you stand up from sitting or lying down. Symptoms include dizziness, fainting (syncope), confusion, or blurred vision.

Patients being admitted to hospital from the community, on any of these 'high risk drugs' should be reviewed by a Doctor or Pharmacist and all staff should be made aware of this risk factor. Table 1.2 shows some of these drugs to be made aware of.

Table 1.2 Drugs which may contribute to falls.

Drug class	Indications	Examples of drugs
Antipsychotics	Psychosis delirium	Haloperidol, Promazine, Trifluoperazine, Quetiapine, Olanzapine, Prochlorperazine. Risperidone
Antidepressants	Mood	Amitriptyline, Trazodone, Fluoxetine, Citalopram. Paroxetine, Sertraline
Hypnotics (sedatives)	Insomnia	Zopiclone, Zolpidem
Benzodiazepines Hypnotics (sedatives)	Insomnia, agitation	Diazepam, Lorazepam, Temazepam, Nitrazepam
Anti-hypertensives	High blood pressure	Ramipril, Lisinopril, Perindopril, Valsartan, Hydralazine, Bisoprolol, Atenolol, Propranolol
Antidiabetics	Diabetes	Glibenclamide, Glipizide, Metformin, Sitagliptin
Opiates	Pain	Codeine, Tramadol, Morphine, Fentanyl, Buprenorphine, Oxycodone
Diuretics	Heart failure, fluid overload, hypertension	Bendroflumethiazide, Furosemide, Bumetanide, Amiloride
Nitrates	Cardiovascular disease	Isosorbide mononitrate, Glyceryltrinitrate (GTN) Nicorandil
Parkinson's Medication	Parkinson's disease	Co-Beneldopa, Co-Careldopa, Selegline Hydrochloride, Pramipexole
Non-steroidal anti-inflammatory drug (NSAIDS)	Pain, inflammation	Ibuprofen, Naproxen, Diclofenac

Drug class	Indications	Examples of drugs
Antimuscarinics (anticholinergics)	These are mentioned in other classes, e.g. for urinary incontinence	Procyclidine, Oxybutynin, Tolterodine, Amitriptyline
Aminoglycosides	Infection	Vancomycin, Gentamicin
Antihistamines	Allergies, itch	Chlorphenamine, Hydralazine, Cetirizine

ADMINISTERING DRUGS SAFELY

Drug Administration Competence

Many hospitals have drug administration competencies for staff to 'prove' that they are competent in the clinical skill of drug administration. Only when these competencies have been signed off can a nurse administer medications alone. Also, the student in healthcare, i.e. Registered nurse, Nursing Associate, etc. will need to be signed off in their medicines management competencies as part of their pre-reg training. Appendix 1 shows an adaption of a typical section of post-reg medicines management competencies.

Calculations Competence

Also, in order to be able to administer intravenous medications, qualified staff are required to pass a drug calculations test to prove mathematical ability, as poor mathematical skills have been indicated in medication errors with the misplacement of the decimal point leading to a tenfold error overdosing or underdosing. Many healthcare environments also set calculation tests during the interview stage.

Activity 1.4 shows a sample question of the sort that you may be expected to answer in one of these tests. Don't worry if your reaction to answering these questions is 😮 we'll go through this in Chapter 4.

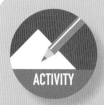

Activity 1.4

Drug calculations sample question.

A drug is presented as 5 g in 500 ml A patient weighing 70 kg is prescribed 10 mg/kg/h of the drug.

1 How many milligrammes per hour of the drug does the patient need?
2 How many millilitres per hour do you set the infusion pump?

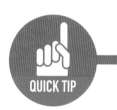

QUICK TIP

To first work out how much of the drug the patient requires according to their body weight we use the formula weight (kg) × dose, and then using the formula:

$$\text{Volume of drug to be given} = \frac{\text{what you want}}{\text{what you've got}} \times \text{volume}$$

But remember to keep the decimal units the same throughout the formula.

Reports and Safety Alerts

In order to alert health carers of the problems around drug administration, the Department of Health and National Safety Patient Agency (NPSA) issue reports and safety alerts, perhaps when mistakes have been made for shared awareness:

- Problems with missed doses,
- Promoting safer use/monitoring of patients on anticoagulant therapy (e.g. warfarin for deep-vein thrombosis [DVT]),

- Promoting safer measurement and administration of liquid medicines,
- Promoting safer use of injectable medicines,
- Safer practice with epidural injections and infusions.

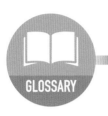

Department of Health
The government department responsible for health regulation and policy in the United Kingdom.

Venous thromboembolism (VTE)
A medical condition including DVT, whereby a blood clot forms inside a vein, and pulmonary embolism (PE), whereby part of the DVT breaks off and travels to the lungs, blocking the blood flow.

Improving Medication Safety

The NPSA produced seven key actions to improve medication safety which are still relevant today (Table 1.3).

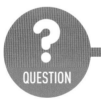

Question 1.5   Why do you think it is important that we know not just what medications the patients are allergic to, but also what foodstuffs?

Patient Self-Administration of Medication

Health carers often take over the medication care of in-patients with diabetes and mess up their blood sugars by not being able to deliver their insulin and other medications at the correct times. Patients with Parkinson's disease also have strict regimes and we may again fail to deliver their medications on time, with profound effects on their independence and wellbeing. Many hospitals now have secure boxes at the bedside for patients to store their medication and allow them to self-medicate.

Table 1.3 Seven key actions to improve medication safety.

Increase reporting	**Increase reporting and identify actions against local risks by way of an annual medication report: clinical risk.**
Implement NPSA safer medication practice recommendations	**Implement NPSA recommendations – audit safer medication practice – includes alerts on anticoagulants, injectable medications, and wrong-route errors.**
Improve staff skills and competencies	**Improve skills: preceptorship competencies will help nurses to work towards the required level of competence.**
Minimise dosing errors	**Minimise errors: information, training, and tools to make calculations easier.**
Ensure medicines are not omitted	**It also can be linked with neglect when medications are not given. The NPSA reviews medicine storage and medication supply chains.**
Ensure medicines are given to the correct patient	**Ensure correct medications with correct patient – improve packaging and labelling of medicines – support local systems that make it harder for staff to select the wrong medicine.**
Document patient's medicine allergy status	**Document: improve recording of patient's allergy status.**

Source: Department of Health (2007).

Remember that not all patients have the ability to do this; for example, patients with dementia or those too ill to administer their own medication. But please remember, patients with dementia may have windows of opportunity whereby they can self-medicate. As with all health care, this aspect of their care must be monitored frequently. Many patients in the community have their medication distributed by their pharmacist into 'dosset' boxes, boxes that have timed sections or partitioned by morning, afternoon, or evening, in order for them to take their medication.

Focus on the Task in Hand: Do Not Get Distracted

Many wards and clinical areas have notices on drug trolleys stating Do Not Disturb While Administering Drugs. This enables the member of staff to concentrate on the task in hand. Some institutions have trialled the wearing of tabards in clinical areas for staff administering drugs, alerting others in the area not to disturb them.

Vicarious Liability

Question 1.6   What does vicarious liability mean?

We all need to comply with our Policies and Procedures, whether we work in a hospital, clinic, or the community setting.

Procedure for Administering Medication

So, when administering medications, what is the correct procedure? The person administering a drug before giving it will:

1   Check the identity of the patient,
2   Check for any recorded allergy/sensitivity,
3   Check the drug name, dose form, strength, date, and time,
4   Check the route of administration,
5   Check for any additional instructions, including safety considerations,
6   Check the drug has not already been administered,
7   Check the drug label against the prescription,
8   Check the expiry date of the drug on the label,
9   Calculate the dose if appropriate.

Prescriptions should be written in black pen, clearly, using no drug trade names, and the member of staff should not be distracted from the task in hand. Medical gases should also be prescribed (except in emergency situations).

When administering medications, we should adhere to the so-called five rights:

- Right medicine,
- Right dose,
- Right route,
- Right patient,
- Right time.

The procedure for checking the patient's name, name band, and prescription chart is referred to as the three-point check.

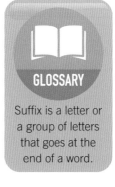

GLOSSARY

Suffix is a letter or a group of letters that goes at the end of a word.

Commonly Used Medicine Name Suffixes

As our knowledge of medicines increase, we will begin to see patterns of drug names related to their drug class, or medicine name suffixes. We can see some of these below in Table 1.4:

Table 1.4 Medicine name suffixes.

Suffix	Medication family or class	Examples of drugs	Indications for use
• mab	Monoclonal antibodies	Trastuzumab Pertvzumab Pembrolizumab	Breast cancer Breast cancer Melanoma
• olol	b-Blockers	Propranolol Bisoprolol Timolol Maleate	Hypertension Adjunct in heart failure Angina
• sartan	Angiotensin receptor antagonists	Valsartan Telmisartan Irbesartan	Hypertension Hypertension Hypertension
• pril	Angotensin-converting Enzyme inhibitors	Lisinopril Ramipril Quinapril	Hypertension Hypertension Hypertension
• cillin	Penicillin antibiotics	Ampicillin Amoxicillin Benzylpenicillin	Susceptible infections e.g. bronchitis Susceptible infections e.g. sinusitis Mild to moderate bacterial infections e.g. pneumonia
• sone	Corticosteroids	Prednisone Dexamethasone Hydrocortisone	Rheumatoid arthritis Cerebral oedema Anaphylaxis

Finally

Before administering any drug to any patient:

- Go through the procedural steps for administering medication in your mind,
- Go through the five rights,
- Know your patient,
- Know the drug and its contraindications.

Lastly, do not cut corners. We all have time constraints, but we must always adhere to the Code of Conduct of the Nursing and Midwifery Council (2015) in order to achieve safe, effective, and professional care for our patients.

TEST YOUR KNOWLEDGE

1   What does STAT mean?
2   What does PRN mean?
3   What are the four parts of the medication process?
4   What route of administration is referred to if you see INH on a prescription chart?
5   A drug is presented as 1 g in 100 ml. A patient weighing 90 kg is prescribed 20 mg/kg/h of the drug.
     (a)   How many milligrammes per hour of the drug does the patient require?
     (b)   For how many millilitres per hour do you set the infusion pump?
6   What are the five rights in regard to drug administration?
7   How many medication errors are there estimated to be in the NHS per annum?
8   According to the BNF, children have been classified into four groups/What are they?
9   If you saw the drug suffix 'olol' what medication class do these drugs belong to?
10   What does ADME stand for?

KEY POINTS

- Latin abbreviations used in drug administration.
- Using your professional judgement.
- The medication process.
- The routes of drug administration.
- Examples of drug administration competencies to be signed off during placements.
- Looking at the front sheet of the prescription chart.
- Improving medication safety factors.
- The procedure for the administration of medicines.

WEB RESOURCES

BNF for Adults: www.bnf.nice.org.uk
BNF for Children: www.bnfc.nice.org.uk
Electronic Medicines Compendium: www.medicines.org.uk/emc
NMC: www.nmc.uk.org
Government publications:
www.gov.uk/government/publications/public-spending-statistics
www.legislation.gov.uk
www.england.nhs.uk/patient-safety/national-medicines-safety-programme
www.gov.uk/government/publications/medication-errors-short-life-working-group-report
www.npsa.org.uk
www.gov.uk/government/publications/the-national-patient-safety-agency-annual-report-and-account
www.england.hns.uk/patient-safety/national-medicines-safety-agency-7-key-actions-to-improve-mrdication-safety
Electronic Medicines Compendium: www.medicines.org.uk
National Patient Safety Agency: www.npsa.nhs.uk

REFERENCE

The Royal Marsden Manual of Clinical Nursing Procedure (2020) (eds.Sara Lister, *Justine Hofland, and Hayley Grafton.* 10. Wiley
NMC (2015) The Code. Professional Standards of Practice and Behaviour for Nurses, Midwives, and Nursing Associates. London. www.nmc.org.uk

Chapter 2

· ·

PHARMACOKINETICS AND PHARMACODYNAMICS

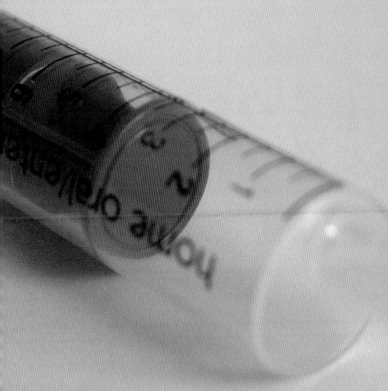

Medicine Management Skills for Nurses, Second Edition. Claire Boyd.
© 2022 John Wiley & Sons Ltd. Published 2022 by John Wiley & Sons Ltd.

LEARNING OUTCOMES

By the end of this chapter you will have an understanding of the general principles of pharmacokinetics and pharmacodynamics, and of adverse drug reactions (ADR) and interactions, including anaphylaxis.

Pharmacodynamics can be defined as what the *drug* does to the *body*: the interaction of the drug within the cell to produce biochemical or physiological changes in the body.

In some cases, the medicine will be used to replace a deficiency, such as:

* thyroxine (given orally): taken for hypothyroidism,
* insulin (given subcutaneously): taken for diabetes mellitus,
* hydroxocobalamin (given intramuscularly): taken for pernicious anaemia,
* ferrous salts (given orally): taken for iron deficiency,
* electrolytes (given orally in aqueous solution): taken for severe cases of diarrhoea.

Pharmacokinetics is the *handling of a drug* in the *body*, or, put another way, what the body does to the medicine. For a drug to be effective it needs to be administered via a suitable route, **absorbed** through the skin, bronchi, or gastrointestinal tract and **distributed** to the site of action, usually via the circulation. The medication will then be **metabolised** or broken down in order to be removed or **excreted** from the body. Some drugs may be eliminated without being metabolised.

The processes that occur after a drug is administered can be broken down into four areas which are; Absorption, Distribution, Metabolism, and Excretion (known as **ADME**). Let's look at these individually, starting with absorption.

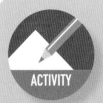

Activity 2.1

From the above paragraph, what four things do you think pharmacokinetics deals with?

ABSORPTION

I once informed a colleague that our new patient had been prescribed diclofenac sodium by the medic, but this patient had stated on admission that non-steroidal antiinflammatory drugs (or NSAIDs) caused him gastrointestinal problems. I was wrongly told that this was 'OK, as we'll give it via the rectum'. It was obvious that this nurse did not fully understand pharmacokinetic concepts. The drug in question would still need to go through the process of absorption and be distributed via the systemic circulation.

Routes of Absorption

- Enteral (Figure 2.1), such as the oral or sublingual routes.

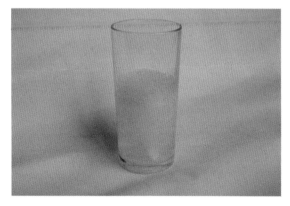

Figure 2.1 How a drug may be given by the enteral route of absorption.

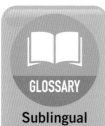

- Parenteral (Figure 2.2), such as by injection and other non-oral routes (for example, the rectum).

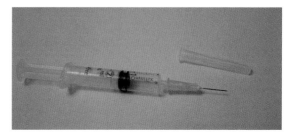

Figure 2.2 How a drug may be given by the parenteral route of absorption.

- Topical (Figure 2.3), such as transdermal or inhalation.

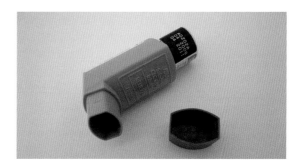

Figure 2.3 How a drug may be given by the inhalation route of absorption.

So, absorption is the movement of the drug from the administration site to the systemic circulation.

The most common means of drug administration is the oral route and both the **amount** absorbed and the **rate** of absorption are determined by the following key factors:

- The physical nature of the dosage form,
- The presence of food (or not) in the stomach,
- The composition of the gastrointestinal contents,
- The gastric or intestinal pH,
- Mesenteric blood flow,
- Concurrent administration with other drugs.

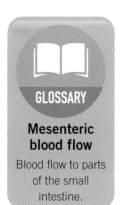

Bioavailability

Bioavailability is the proportion of the administered drug that reaches the systemic circulation. It refers to the amount of drug available for distribution to the intended site of action.

Drugs administered by the intravenous (IV) route are considered to have 100% bioavailability. Drugs administered via the oral route tend not to have high bioavailability, so are usually prescribed at higher doses than parenterally administered drugs. For example, propranolol (a beta-blocker) may be prescribed orally in doses of 40 mg and above. The equivalent IV dose is 1 mg/ml.

DRUG DISTRIBUTION

When a drug enters the bloodstream, it is rapidly diluted and transported around the body. Movement from the blood to the tissues of the body is influenced by a number of key factors. One of these is the plasma proteins, which can bind many drugs. Only the unbound fraction of the drug is free to move from the bloodstream into tissues to exert a pharmacological effect.

The central nervous system is predominantly surrounded by a specialised membrane, known as the **blood–brain barrier**, which is highly selective for lipid-soluble drugs. For example, penicillins diffuse well in body tissues and fluids but penetration into the cerebrospinal fluid is generally poor. An example of the blood–brain barrier can be seen in the treatment for Parkinson's disease. Dopamine does not cross the blood–brain barrier and is therefore administered as a precursor, levodopa. Levodopa is administered, absorbed, crosses the blood–brain barrier and is broken down to dopamine by the enzyme dopa decarboxylase. Bingo!

During pregnancy the **placenta** also provides a barrier between mother and foetus. Some drugs cross it relatively easily (such as chlorpromazine and morphine), whereas others (such as suxamethonium chloride – a neuromuscular blocker) do not.

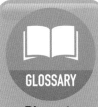

DRUG METABOLISM

Drugs that are taken orally dissolve in gastric fluid and to diffuse across membranes they must be lipid-soluble. The higher the solubility in lipids, the more rapidly will the drug diffuse into the tissues. The main site of drug metabolism is the liver, but other tissues may also metabolise drugs, such as the:

- Lungs,
- Kidneys,
- Blood,
- Intestine.

DRUG EXCRETION

Most drugs are excreted by the kidneys. The rate of excretion varies greatly: some are excreted within the hour whereas some take days or even weeks. Individuals with renal impairment may excrete certain drugs more slowly. This will have important consequences if the usual dose is not reduced as plasma levels of the drug will rise, producing possible toxic effects.

Therapeutic Serum Levels

It is important to take all medication at the correct intervals, as prescribed.

This is to maintain therapeutic serum levels, which the Scientists have worked out for each drug when developing the drug. This is why some tablets are 500 or 2 mg or 1 g, etc. In other words, what the dose needs to be to 'hit the spot'. Below shows what happens to the therapeutic serum levels when we take a medicine:

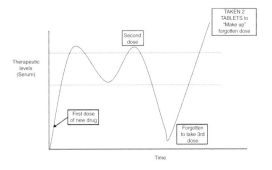

1   We take the first dose of a medicine, which hits the therapeutic level.
2   We take the second dose of our new medicine, to maintain the therapeutic level.
3   We then forget to take the third dose of our medication and our blood serum level for the medicine falls below the therapeutic serum level.
4   We decide to take two doses of the new medicine to make up for forgetting to take it earlier. **STOP!** This should never be done. Seek advice from a Pharmacist, Doctor, or from the National Health Service (NHS) helpline (call 111). Taking two tablets at once can cause toxicity and potential harm.

DRUG INTERACTIONS

Drug interactions occur when two or more drugs react with each other, which can cause unexpected side effects or may even increase the action of a drug. Some drug interactions can be harmful: a negative drug interaction. Others may be more beneficial, such as that of paracetamol (acetaminophen) and morphine: a positive drug interaction.

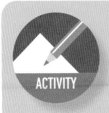

Activity 2.2

ACTIVITY

Why would paracetamol and morphine taken together be said to have a beneficial drug interaction in many cases?

Synergy and Antagonism

When drugs interact and cause an increase in the effects of one or both of the drugs, the interaction is called a synergistic effect. The opposite effect to synergy is termed antagonism. Two drugs are antagonistic when their interaction causes a decrease in the effects of one or both drugs.

Drug Interaction: Underlying Factors

Four of the factors that predispose a person to drug interactions are listed here.

- *Age*: physiological changes occur as we age, and these changes may affect the interaction of drugs. Liver metabolism, kidney function, nerve transmission, and the functioning of bone marrow all decrease with age.
- *Polypharmacy*: the more drugs an individual takes, the more chance that some of them will interact.
- *Genetic factors*: genes code for the enzymes that metabolise drugs. Some genotypic variations decrease or increase the activity of these enzymes.
- *Hepatic or renal diseases*: drugs that are metabolised in the liver and/or eliminated by the kidneys may be altered if these organs are not functioning correctly.

Drug–Food Beverage Interaction

Drugs can also interact with some food and beverages; indeed, alcohol cannot be taken with a lot of medications. Patients who drink alcohol and take paracetamol on a regular basis are at increased risk of developing liver damage. Patients taking oxycodone hydrochloride (an opioid analgesic) may get worse if they eat or drink grapefruit juice. This is because chemicals in grapefruit products may interfere with the enzymes that metabolise (break down) the medication in your system, increasing the potency of the drug to potentially dangerous levels and causing severe side effects. You might want to look at the Complementary Therapy section in Chapter 1, if you skipped this section.

Table 2.1 shows some foods and drugs that are affected by the food's influence on drug metabolism.

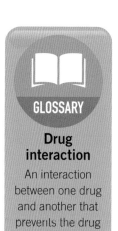

GLOSSARY

Drug interaction

An interaction between one drug and another that prevents the drug from performing as expected.

Drug–Medical Condition Interaction

Existing medical conditions can also present problems when taking certain drugs. For example, if someone has hypertension, harm may be caused by taking a nasal decongestant.

Table 2.1 Foods and the drugs affected due to the influence on drug metabolism.

Food	Drugs affected
Avocado	Warfarin
Grapefruit juice	Nifedipine, nimodipine, carbamazepine, midazolam
Soya	Haloperidol, phenytoin, warfarin
Garlic	Anticoagulants
Ginseng	Warfarin, heparin, aspirin
Ginger	Anticoagulants
Chamomile	Benzodiazepines, barbiturates, and opioids

The Pharmacist

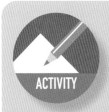

Activity 2.3

Who is the best person/people to speak to if you require information regarding drug interactions?

Most large hospitals wards have a designated pharmacist who visits the ward regularly. It is at this time that they will monitor the prescription charts in the dispensary and on the ward, assessing prescriptions for accuracy, legibility, interactions, and appropriateness of therapy in line with evidence-based clinical practise. In the community information can be sought from the chemist Pharmacist.

Adverse Drug Reactions

An ADR (adverse drug reaction) tends to refer to harm caused by a drug at *normal doses, during normal use*. An ADR is not the same as an allergy, which is an ADR mediated by an immune response.

All medicines undergo a series of clinical trials before they are licensed for use. However, it is often only when a medicine becomes available to millions of people that side effects may become apparent. An adverse drug reaction (often abbreviated to ADR) may be produced by any drug, as no effective medicine is entirely free from side effects.

In the UK it is the **Medicines and Healthcare Products Regulatory Agency** (MHRA) that oversees the medicines we take and ensures that the medical devices we use are safe. The study of ADRs is known as **pharmacovigilance**.

Reporting Adverse Drug Reactions

It may be difficult to establish definitely that a medicine has caused a side effect but, even so, if you suspect that a medicine has caused a reaction it should still be reported. Reporting is carried out by the 'yellow card' scheme in the UK. These yellow cards can be found at the back of copies the *British National Formulary* (or BNF) and forwarded via FREEPOST. They can also be accessed online at www.yellowcard.gov.uk. Further information on how to complete this document can be found on the website.

NOTE: there is a BNF for adults and one specifically for children.

Healthcare professionals can help improve medicines safety by completing this document; by being the Government's eyes and ears. How else will they know that patients are experiencing adverse drug effects? Without reporting side effects, no one will be aware that a medicine is causing problems. Have you heard of the drug thalidomide? This was prescribed for morning sickness in pregnancy and was later found to cause birth defects. It is now licensed for untreated multiple myeloma in patients aged 65 years and over.

Patients can also complete yellow cards, which can be found in general practitioner (GP) surgeries and pharmacies, as well as at the website given above.

The MHRA can establish whether a drug's risk is 'common' or 'serious' and then decide what action to take. The MHRA rarely takes a medicine off the market, but if the risk associated with a medicine outweighs its benefit, then this step may be taken. The MHRA looks at:

- The potential risks associated with the side effects of the medicine, and
- The risk to the patient if the condition is not treated.

Since 1964, when the yellow card scheme was set up, over 600 000 UK yellow cards have been submitted.

ANAPHYLAXIS

DID YOU KNOW?

Children are more likely to have an allergic reaction to food stuffs e.g. peanuts, bananas
   Adults are more likely to have a reaction to a medication e.g. penicillin, NSAIDs

Anaphylaxis is an extreme adverse allergic reaction to a trigger antigen and can be triggered by drugs, food items, latex, injected venom, and basically anything that a person may be allergic to. The body recognizes the antigen as a foreign invader and produces antibodies to fight it. It is caused when the immune system releases a flood of chemicals that can cause the body to go into shock whereby the blood pressure drops suddenly and the airways narrow. A full A – E assessment of the individual should be performed, and in the case of anaphylaxis, you will observe:

Airway – Difficulty breathing and swallowing, sensation of throat closing over, hoarse voice
Breathing – Shortness of voice, increased respiratory rate, wheeze
Circulation – Signs of shock (pale and calmy), increased pulse rate (tachycardia), weak pulse, low blood pressure (hypotension)

Disability – Anxiety, panic, decreased conscious level, dizziness, Nausea, and vomiting

Exposure – Erythema (red skin rash), urticaria (blisters on skin), angioedema (swelling around eyelids, lips, and sometimes the mouth and throat)

The Resuscitation Council (UK) are responsible for setting central standards for cardiopulmonary resuscitation; as a healthcare professional you will be or have already been introduced to the algorithm for resuscitation (www.resus.org.uk). It is important you are fully conversant with this. As a general rule, the actions to take are as follows:

A – E assessment	Look for airway or breathing problems and/or circulatory problems. Also skin changes
Call for help	Lie patient flat, with legs raised
Administer adrenalin	IM Adult: 500 mg/0.5 ml Children > 12 yr old 500 mg = 0.5 ml Children 6–12 yr old 300 mg = 0.3 ml Children < 6 yr old 150 mg = 0.15 ml Repeat after 5 min if no change to patients condition
Establish airway Administer high flow oxygen Administer IV fluids Administer chlorphenamine Administer hydrocortisone	Monitor pulse oximetry Perform ECG Monitor blood pressure

Did you ever wonder why we administer adrenaline (epinephrine) in anaphylaxis? How does it reverse the anaphylaxis effects?

Adrenaline is administered due to the fact that during anaphylaxis, the blood vessels 'leak,' the bronchial tissues swell, and the blood pressure drops, causing the choking and collapse. Adrenaline acts quickly to:

- Constrict blood vessels
- Relax smooth muscles in the lungs to improve breathing
- Stimulates the hearts contractility
- Helps to stop the swelling around the face and lips (angio-oedema)

Other drugs we may administer during an anaphylaxis are Salbutamol to aid bronchial dilation, Chlorphenamine – an antihistamine, Hydrocortisone – an anti-inflammatory, and IV fluids. It is always important to read the Patient Information Leaflet (PIL) that comes with all drugs to ascertain whether the drug contains anything someone may be allergic to.

The Patient Information Leaflet

All medicines have a PIL that gives instructions on how to take the medicine, its side effects and a list of all ingredients. Let's look at one of these in detail for a drug prescribed for breast cancer.

Exemestane, 25 mg Coated Tablets

The information sheet first tells us that this drug is called Aromasin and that it belongs to a group of medicines known as aromatase inhibitors that interfere with a substance called aromatase, which is needed to make the female hormone oestrogen. It then says that reducing the oestrogen levels in the body is a way of treating breast cancer.

The leaflet goes into more detail about what the drug is used for. In the next section of the leaflet there is advice on 'Before you take Aromasin' and 'Take Special Care with Aromasin', advising that this drug may lead to a loss of the mineral content of bones, which may decrease their strength.

The leaflet then states that Aromasin should not be taken at the same time as hormone-replacement therapy and that the patient's doctor needs to be informed if the following drugs are being taken, advising caution:

- Rifampicin (an antibiotic),
- Carbamazepine or phenytoin (anticonvulsants used to treat epilepsy),
- St John's wort herbal remedy.

Then there are sections on pregnancy and breast feeding, driving and using machines, and some important information about some of the ingredients and sugar intolerances. Following this there are sections on 'How to take Aromasin' and what to do if you forget to take the drug or take more of the drug than you should. Other sections include 'How To Store Aromasin' and what the drug contains and looks like in the pack.

By far the largest section is on possible side effects, and these include:

Very Common Side Effects

- Difficulty sleeping
- Headache
- Hot flushes
- Feeling sick
- Increased sweating
- Muscle and joint pain
- Tiredness

Common Side Effects

- Loss of appetite
- Depression
- Dizziness
- Carpal tunnel syndrome
- Stomach ache, vomiting, constipation, indigestion, diarrhoea
- Skin rash, hair loss
- Thinning of bones
- Pain, swollen hands and feet

Uncommon Side Effects

- Drowsiness
- Muscle weakness
- Inflammation of the liver: hepatitis may occur

The BNF Side Effects Grading Scheme

The BNF lists side effects in order of frequency, which is described as:

- very common (greater than 1 in 10),
- common (1 in 100 to 1 in 10),
- less commonly (1 in 1000 to 1 in 100),
- rarely (1 in 10000 to 1 in 1000),
- very rarely (less than 1 in 10000),
- frequency not known.

Examples of Some Adverse Effects

You should get used to looking up medicines, ready for when you start going on drug rounds or become involved with the administration of drugs. If you look through the BNF, and look at the drugs, you will see a section entitled Side effects. It is the nurse's responsibility to have knowledge of these whenever administering prescribed medications, as well as the Cautions and Contraindications. Table 2.2 shows just a very small selection of drugs and some of their reported side effects. You may already be familiar with some of these drugs; others you may wish to look up.

Table 2.2 A selection of drugs and some of their reported side effects.

Drug	Potential side effects
Aspirin (acetylsalicylic acid)	Bronchospasm, gastro-intestinal irritation, increased bleeding time
Ampicillin (penicillin)	Nausea, vomiting, diarrhoea, rashes
Phenobarbital (for control of epilepsy)	Hepatitis, cholestasis, hypotension, respiratory depression, behavioural disturbances
Ispaghula husk (bulk-forming laxative)	Flatulence, abdominal distension, gastrointestinal obstruction or impaction

(Continued)

Table 2.2 (*Continued*)

Drug	Potential side effects
Gentamicin (aminoglycoside)	Vestibular and auditory damage, nephrotoxicity, nausea, vomiting, rash, blood disorders
Propofol (intravenous anaesthetic)	Hypotension, tachycardia, flushing, transient apnoea, hyperventilation, coughing, hiccups (during induction)
Paracetamol (acetaminophen)	Malaise, skin reactions, hepatotoxic in high doses
Diazepam (anxiolytic)	Drowsiness and light-headedness the next day, confusion and ataxia (especially in the elderly), amnesia, dependence, dysarthria, muscle weakness, paradoxical increase in aggression
Metoclopramide hydrochloride (antiemetic)	Extrapyramidal effects (especially in children and young adults), anxiety, confusion, drowsiness, restlessness, diarrhoea, depression
Sumatriptan (antimigraine drug)	Sensations of tingling, heat, heaviness, pressure, or tightness of any part of the body (including the throat and chest), drowsiness, transient increase in blood pressure
Ipratropium bromide spray (antimuscarinic bronchodilator)	Epistaxis, nasal dryness, and irritation; less frequently: nausea, headache, and pharyngitis

TEST YOUR KNOWLEDGE

Below are the details of six patients. See if you can work out whether the patient's clinical features are the result of an adverse reaction or something else. **Remember**: an ADR tends to refer to harm caused by a drug at normal doses, during normal use.

1   Betty Leaman is prescribed a litre of 5% glucose with 20 mmol of potassium chloride over eight hours. You put up the IV infusion, by gravity feed as no pumps are available, set the rate and leave the patient with her visitors, who have just arrived. The visitors ask if they can take Betty out for a short time to the local pub 'to cheer her up'. You explain this is not possible as Betty

has an infusion running that has been prescribed to run over eight hours. Two hours later one of the visitors comes to you saying that the infusion has finished, but Betty is uncomfortable and feeling unwell. When you go to assess Betty, you find her to be restless, dyspnoeic, and tachycardic. Is this an ADR?

2   Jenny Heller is 28 years of age. Jenny gave birth to a beautiful baby daughter eight weeks ago. She is known to be hypertensive and been prescribed bromocriptine 2.5 mg tablets for 3 days, then 2.5 mg twice daily for 14 days, for the suppression of lactation. Jenny has read the patient information sheet and queries whether it is OK to take this medication because it states that this drug should not be used in postpartum women with high blood pressure as this is a contra-indication. Her GP asks her when she got her PhD and tells her that he knows best. Jenny takes the medication but experiences nausea, headache, dizziness, and dyskinesia. Is this an ADR?

3   Daisy Bovan is 72 years of age and has been experiencing neurogenic bladder instability resulting in urinary incontinence. Her GP has prescribed oxybutynin hydrochloride 2.5 mg tablets twice a day. Daisy takes the medication as prescribed but starts complaining of feeling 'hot' and faint. The GP checks the prescription, and the prescription is correct, but side effects are reported as being 'reduced sweating leading to heat sensations and fainting in hot environments'. Is this an ADR?

4   Michelle Proser is a student nurse and is usually quite fit and well apart from her pernicious anaemia. Michelle has been prescribed intramuscular injections of hydroxocobalamin (administered by a practice nurse). The dose Michelle has been prescribed is 1 mg/ml every three months. This is the correct prescription. Not long after receiving her injection Michelle starts complaining of feeling nauseous and having a headache. One of her colleagues looks this up in the BNF and finds that it is a side effect of the drug. Is this an ADR?

5 Peter Flavia is two years old and weighs 14 kg. He has been prescribed Benzylpenicillin 50 mg/kg every six hours (weight × dose = 14 × 50 = 700 mg). This is to be administered by intermittent intravenous infusion in sodium chloride 0.9% given over 30 minutes. Within a very short time span Peter becomes fractious and angioedema is noticed to his facial and neck area. His voice sounds husky. The prescription is correct. Is this an ADR?

6 Sophie Davis has respiratory distress syndrome. Sophie is 10 years old and weighs 30 kg. Furosemide 5 mg/kg has been prescribed by slow intravenous injection (weight × dose = 30 × 5 = 150 mg). Shortly after administration, Sophie's observations show hypotension. Blood tests show hyponatraemia. Sophie is complaining of deafness. Is this an ADR?

KEY POINTS

- The principles of pharmacodynamics.
- The principles of pharmacokinetics.
- The principles of bioavailability.
- Underlying factors affecting drug interactions.
- Understanding anaphylaxis
- How to report ADRs.
- Looking at PILs.

WEB RESOURCES

Yellow Card Scheme: www.yellowcard.mhra.gov.uk
BNF: www.bnf.nice.org.uk
Medicines and Healthcare Products Regulatory Agency: www.mhra.gov.uk
Resus Council: www.resus.org.uk
Anaphylaxis: www.nhs.uk/conditions/anaphylaxis/
NHS Helpline: www.111.nhs.uk
Electronic Medicines Compendium: www.medicines.org.uk

Chapter 3
· ·
DRUGS AND MEDICINES

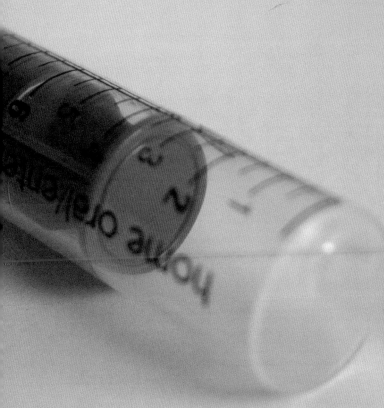

LEARNING OUTCOMES

By the end of this chapter you will have an understanding of the general principles of drugs and medicines including legislation and standards relating to medicines management.

WHAT'S THE DIFFERENCE BETWEEN A DRUG AND A MEDICINE?

Drugs are substances that, when taken into the body, affect the structure or function of this living organism.

Medicines can be said to be drugs that are used in the treatment, diagnosis, or prevention of a disease. All medicines have a product licence (PL) number to indicate that they have been licensed for use as a medicine. If a drug does not have a PL number, it cannot be licensed as a medicine.

CATEGORIES OF MEDICINE

Categories of medicine are given in Table 3.1.

Table 3.1 Categories of medicine.

Legal category of medicine	What it means
GSL	General Sales List medicines These are drugs you can buy in small packs (16), such as paracetamol in your local supermarket. Also known as Over the Counter (OTC) medicines
P	Pharmacy medicines Before selling, a pharmacist has to be in the local vicinity. These medicines may cause harm. For drugs such as sumatriptan, a pharmacist has to authorise the sale as an extra intervention and ask a few questions, such as 'have you taken this drug before?'
POM	Prescription-Only Medicines These drugs have to be prescribed and cannot be bought over the counter.

Legal category of medicine	What it means
POM-CD	Prescription-Only Medicines-Controlled Drugs There are five categories of controlled drugs: *Schedule 1* no medical purpose, e.g. cannabis *Schedule 2* most likely to cause harm but has a medical purpose, e.g. MST. Such drugs have to have an audit trial, and a collector and/or receiver has to sign for this type of drug. *Schedule 3* must be entered into a controlled drugs book, e.g. temazepam *Schedule 4*, e.g. diazepam *Schedule 5*, e.g. kaolin and morphine

Prescription Only Medications-Community

In the community, prescription-only medicines (POMs) are prescription medicines, which a general practitioner (GP) can prescribe using a prescription form. Written prescriptions can be kept for up to six months before they must be taken to a pharmacist. This period is 28 days for controlled drugs. The front of the written prescription form has the patient's name, age (if under 12 years), medicine name, form, strength, quantity to supply, and dose. It must also have the GP's or prescriber's signature, the date, and GP's or prescriber's stamp.

The back of this form has to be signed by the person collecting the drug from the pharmacist: this is the patient or other person taking responsibility for the medication (such as a parent for a child's prescription).

MEDICATION DIRECTIONS

When we take a prescription from our GP to the local pharmacist the medicines we then receive will have medication directions. Medicine bottles and containers are required *by law* to have a directions label attached. Now you will see where the abbreviations given in Chapter 1 come into play. Some of the instructions you may see on this labelling include:

- One to be taken each day (1 OD),
- One to be taken twice a day (1 BD),

- One to be taken three times a day (1 TDS or 1 TID),
- One to be taken four times a day (1 QDS or 1 QID).

PRESCRIPTIONS

- Drugs that are prescribed every 12 hours (twice a day – BD) such as at 8 a.m. and 8 p.m.
- Drugs that are prescribed every eight hours (three times a day – TDS) such as at 7 a.m., 3 p.m., and 11 p.m.
- Drugs that are prescribed every six hours (four times a day – QDS) such as at 6 a.m., 12 midday, 6 p.m., and 12 midnight.

More Labelling

- One to be taken in the morning (1 OM or 1 mane)
- One to be taken at night (1 ON or 1 nocte)
- One or two to be taken when required (1 or 2 PRN [*pro re nata*])

Question 3.1   Can you remember what PRN means?

- Before food (AC [*ante cibum*])
- With food/after food (CC/PC [*post cibum*])
- As directed (MDU)
- Swallow whole: do not chew
- Apply sparingly.

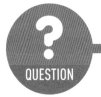

Question 3.2   What do you think the purpose is of AC and CC? And what about 'Do not chew' instructions?

GENERIC PRESCRIBING

Generic prescribing refers to when a drug has been prescribed using it's **non-proprietary name**. This means the chemical or **generic** name, or the approved name of the drug.

This is distinguished from the **proprietary name**, which is a brand name or a trade name.

The following drug is prescribed for asthma and other conditions associated with reversible airway obstruction:

Non-proprietary name	salbutamol (albuterol)
Proprietary name	Ventolin (trade-marked)

Many healthcare environments have their own medicines management policies and usually have a statement along the lines of:

> All drugs prescribed by the approved generic name, written in block capitals (except where prescribing by trade name identifies a particular product where the brand's bioavailability may vary, e.g. specific sustained-release brands). Such products are indicated in the *British National Formulary*.

It should also be noted that the drug should not be given if a prescription is ambiguous or illegible, or an error in the prescription is suspected.

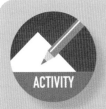

Activity 3.1

You will need to find a copy of the *British National Formulary* or use a computer to go on-line www.bnf.nice.org.uk: What are the proprietary names of these drugs?

Non-proprietary drug name	Proprietary drug name
Nitrazepam (used in insomnia)	
Sodium valproate (used in epilepsy)	
Rivastigmine (used in Alzheimer's disease or Parkinson's disease)	
Pyrimethamine (used in the treatment of malaria)	
Calcium salts/calcium gluconate (used as a calcium supplement)	

Some drugs may be available from a selection of drug companies and may be presented with many different proprietary, trademarked, or generic names, which can become confusing for everyone.

Let me give you an example from paediatric nursing. When giving paracetamol to children or babies, paediatric **oral suspension of paracetamol** is the non-proprietary name we want written on our charts, not the trade name of this preparation, such as Calpol, Disprol, Medinol, Paldesic, or Panadol.

So you can see why it may be best to write up the prescription using the non-proprietary drug name.

TYPES OF MEDICINE

We will be looking at types of medicine in more detail in the following chapters, but let's start with an overview. Table 3.2 lists types of systemic medication, which affect the whole body. Topical medications – usually applied to one site – are listed in Table 3.3.

Some of the other types of injections include: intradermal (into the dermis), intrathecal (into the cerebral spinal fluid), intra-ventricular (into the ventricles of the brain), and intraperitoneal (into the peritoneum body cavity – mainly used in animals by vets)

Table 3.2 Systemic medicines.

Systemic medicines	What are they?
Oral medicines – solid-dose forms	Tablets and capsules Soluble/dispersible/effervescent tablets Lozenges Tablets with an enteric coating Sustained-release tablets and capsules
Oral medicines – liquid-dose forms	Solutions Syrups Suspensions Emulsions
Rectal medicines	Medications for rectal administration
Parenteral medicines (by injection)	Subcutaneous Intravenous Intramuscular Intra-articular Depot injections

Table 3.3 Topical medicines.

Topical medicines	What are they?
Eye, ear, and nasal medications	Drops and sprays
Creams and ointments	Creams tend to be water-based Ointments tend to be more hydrating
Inhalers	Relievers and preventers
Rectal medicines	Suppositories Creams, ointments, and foams Enemas
Vaginal preparations	Pessaries Devices

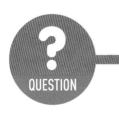

QUESTION

Question 3.3   What are 'depot injections' and intra-articular injections?

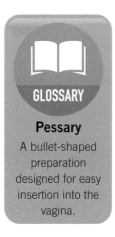

GLOSSARY

Pessary

A bullet-shaped preparation designed for easy insertion into the vagina.

Other routes of administration include dressings (medicated and dry) and transdermal patches, which we will look at in Chapter 8.

The Pharmaceutical industry has also formulated 'wafer-based' versions of medicines, which dissolve rapidly under the tongue. These are aimed at patients who may be unable to swallow tablets – such as migraine sufferers who may experience nausea and vomiting during an episode, so may tolerate rizatriptan wafers. Wafers are also used to treat conditions in which adherence may be an issue, e.g. Olanzapine wafers to treat schizophrenia.

MEDICINE STORAGE

In the hospital setting, drugs may be kept in locked trolleys, lockers or cupboards, cool dry rooms or special drug-only fridges, according to the storage information on the medication. At home we don't have special drug-only fridges, so of course this is only in the professional capacity. One of these special drug fridges will be for vaccines.

VACCINES

As mentioned, some drugs need to be kept in medicine fridges, including many vaccines. The fridge will need to be kept in the very specific temperature range of **2–8 °C**. The fridge is monitored daily and the temperature recorded to make sure that it remains within these parameters. Vaccines may also need to be transported, but in such cases they still need to be kept in the specified temperature range in special transportation cool bags. This process of storage and transfer, keeping the vaccine at the right temperature at every step, is known as the **cold chain**.

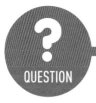

QUESTION

Question 3.4   Why is the cold chain important?

Vaccine fridges need to be dedicated to vaccines and no food or specimens should be put in them. It is also very important to safeguard the electricity supply of such fridges as if the stored vaccines fall out of the cold chain range they are ruined and must not be used. The fridge should only ever be 50% full. The fridge should be defrosted and calibrated regularly, and a back-up system should be available in the event of a fridge failing.

To record the daily details the maximum, minimum, and current temperatures are documented. More information around vaccines, and how they are produced, can be seen in Chapter 6.

LEGISLATION

Next we will look at just some of the legislation around medicines management.

Medicines Act 1968

This Act was the first comprehensive legislation on medicines in the UK. The Act provides a framework for the manufacture, licensing, prescription, supply, and administration of medicines. It is this Act that classifies medicines into the categories of POMs, Pharmacy medicines, and General sales list medicines (GSL).

Misuse of Drugs Act 1971

This Act covers the legislation surrounding the prescription, supply, storage, and administration of medicines. It also prohibits certain activities in relation to the manufacture, supply, and possession of drugs. Drugs are placed in one of three classes depending on their harmfulness if misused.

Class A includes morphine, Fentanyl, Lysergide (LSD), and Pethidine

Class B includes barbiturates, Cannabis, Codeine Phosphate, and Dihydrocodeine

Class C includes Tramadol hydrochloride, anabolic steroids, Gabapentin, and Zopicione

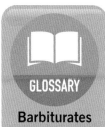

GLOSSARY

Barbiturates

A drug that acts as a central nervous system depressant, e.g. anxiolytics, hypnotics, and anticonvulsants.

The Misuse of Drugs Regulations 2001

Preparations that are subject to the prescription requirements of the Misuse of Drugs Regulations 2001 can be recognised by the symbol CD, meaning controlled drug. These regulations define the classes of persons who are authorised to supply and possess controlled drugs while acting in their professional capacities. In the regulations, the drugs are divided into five schedules, with each specifying the requirements governing such activities as import, export, production, supply, possession, prescribing, and record-keeping which apply to them.

Schedule 1   Possession and supply prohibited unless under Home Office rule, deemed to have no medicinal use. Includes drugs such as hallucinogenics, lysergide (LSD), and ecstasy-type substances. A controlled-drug register must be kept.

Schedule 2   Subject to full controlled drug requirements relating to prescriptions, safe custody, the need to keep registers, etc. Controlled drugs; includes diamorphine hydrochloride (heroin), morphine, pethidine hydrochloride, oxycodone, and cocaine.

Schedule 3   Subject to special prescription requirements and safe custody requirements. Register does not need to be kept. Invoices to be retained for two years. Includes drugs such as buprenorphine, midazolam, temazepam, and tramadol hydrochloride.

Schedule 4   Subject to minimal control. Register does not need to be kept. Part 1 includes benzodiazepines
Part 2 includes Androgenic and anabolic steroids

Schedule 5   Includes preparations of certain controlled drugs (such as codeine and morphine), which due to their low strength are exempt from virtually all CD requirements other than retention of invoices for two years.

Misuse of Drugs (Supply to Addicts) Regulations 1997

This Regulation requires that only Medical Practitioners who hold a special licence issued by the Home Secretary (or Scottish Government Chief Medical Officer) may prescribe, administer, or supply diamorphine hydrochloride, dipipanone, or cocaine for the treatment of drug addition.

Misuse of Drugs (Prescription and Control of Supply of Cannabis for Medical Use) Regulations 2018

Some cannabis-based products have now been made available on prescription as medicinal cannabis under specified therapeutic indications:

1 Spasticity associated with multiple sclerosis resistant to all standard therapies and interventions (Nabiximols).
2 Intractable nausea and vomiting associated with chemotherapy, despite the use of standard anti-emetic regimes (Nabilone).
3 Severe, refractory epilepsy that has failed to respond to standard anticonvulsant medications (Epidyolex).

EC Directive 92/27/EEC

This directive outlines the requirements for the labelling of medicines and for the format of the user leaflets that are supplied with patient packs of medicines. It should be noted, **the UK left the European Union in January 2021.**

The Health Act 2006

This Act informs us that within practice, healthcare workers are governed by something called Standard Operating Procedures (SOPs). In regard to CDs, the SOP will specify who can order CDs for the clinical area, the process to follow, who can transport them to the clinical area and the designated personnel who can receive and enter into the CD register. Each employer is required to appoint an accountable officer – someone not involved in this process.

Nursing Associates will need to check with their health-setting local policy as arrangements differ from organisation to organisation.

The Human Medicines Regulations 2012

This legislation sought to simplify medicines management. An example of this is that anyone can administer certain life-saving medications in emergency situations in order to save a life. The most obvious example of this is adrenaline 1:1000 IM in the case of someone experiencing anaphylaxis.

Health and Safety Act 1974

This Act includes the reporting of accidents and incidences, including:

- **Near misses** – example: about to administer a medicine to the wrong patient.
- **Serious adverse events** – example: Giving the wrong medicine to a patient and they suffer a serious adverse reaction.
- **Never events** – example: a mistake that should never have happened such as administering penicillin to a patient with a known allergy to penicillin and the patient dies.
- **Critical and major incidents** – example: A hospital having to close due to an over-run of pandemic patients.

This Act also covers the disposal of sharps (i.e. injection needles).

I imagine many of you thought that you had finished reading all the legislation stuff, but there's more! It really is important to have an overview of Acts of Parliament for your understanding for the safe administration of medicines, whether you are a student, seasoned health-care professional, or someone returning to practice.

ADMINISTRATION OF DRUGS TO PATIENTS WHO REFUSE TREATMENT

Medicines, as with all forms of treatment, must only be administered with the patient's consent. In the main this is implied by the fact that *the patient* takes the prescribed medication. The only situation where medications may be administered without the patient's consent is under the Mental Health Act 1983.

DID YOU KNOW?

Someone stole my anti-depressants. Well, I hope they're happy now! LOL

Sorry, just thought after all that legislation, we needed something to lighten the mood.

Nursing Standards for Administration of Medicines

Nurses previously adhered to the Nursing and Midwifery Council's *Standards for Medicines Management* (2008); **These were withdrawn on 28 January 2019.**

Nurses, Midwives, and Nursing Associates still adhere to the Code of Professional Standards of Practice and Behaviour (2018), whereby we:

- Prioritise people
- Practise effectively
- Preserve safety
- Promote professionalism and trust.

The Royal College of Nursing and the Royal Pharmaceutical Society have issued 'Professional Guidance on the Administration of Medicines in Healthcare Settings' January 2019. Section 1 of this document informs us that:

> 3. *Medicines are administered in accordance with a prescription, Patient Specific Direction (PSD), Patient Group Direction or other relevant exemption specified in the Human Medicines Regulations 2012. Medicines that are not POMs may be administered according to a locally agreed homely remedy protocol.*

Section 7 of this guidance informs us:

7. Registered healthcare professionals who administer medicines, or when appropriate delegate the administration of medicines are accountable for their actions, non-actions and omissions and exercise professionalism and professional judgement at all times.

WHAT IS ARE PATIENT SPECIFIC AND PATIENT GROUP DIRECTIONS?

PSD: An instruction from a doctor, dentist, or other independent prescriber for a medicine to be supplied or administered to a named patient after the prescriber has assessed that patient on an individual basis, e.g. written direction in patients notes or in-patient chart.

Patient Group Direction (PGD): A written direct that allows the supply and/or administration of a specific medicine or medicines by named authorized health professionals, to a well-defined group of patients requiring treatment of a specific condition.

Putting this into practice, drugs such as adrenaline may need to be given and the PGD allows the nurse to administer this drug without an individual prescription. The PGD contains a list of others who sign this document to state that the drug can be given. Very often clauses are attached, such as that the staff administering the medication must be up to date with their resuscitation training.

The Nursing and Midwifery Council (NMC) have also issued Standards of Proficiency for Registered Nurses (2018) whereby Section 4.14 and 4.15 are particularly relevant:

4.14 *Understand the principles of safe and effective administration and optimisation of medicines in accordance with local and national policies and demonstrate proficiency and accuracy when calculating dosages of prescribed medicines.*

In other words, read the policies and pass your calculations tests!

4.15 *Demonstrate knowledge of pharmacology and the ability to recognise the effects of medicines, allergies, drug sensitivities, side-effects, contraindications, incompatibilities, adverse reactions, prescribing errors, and the impact of polypharmacy and over-the-counter medication usage.*

In other words, pass your medicines competencies (and read this book)!

Apprenticeship Standard for Nursing Associates

The Nursing Associate is part of the Apprenticeship scheme: Standard ST0827 sets out the occupational duties, with the skills, knowledge, and behaviours outlined in order to obtain an accredited award approved by the NMC and to gain registration onto the nursing register. Within its requirements, it specifies for the safe and effective administration and optimisation of medicines in accordance with local and National policies.

In other words, read the policies and procedures!

Unlicensed Medicines

There are clinical situations when the use of unlicensed medicines or use of medicines outside the term of the licence (known as 'off-label') may be judged by the prescriber to be in the best interest of the patient on the basis of available evidence. Such practice is particularly common in certain areas of medicine. An example of this is in paediatrics whereby drugs have been developed for adults only, so when used for children they are being used off-label or are unlicensed.

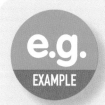

Let me show you an example

EXAMPLE

Paracetamol unlicensed use: Paracetamol oral suspension 500 mg/5 ml is not licensed for use in children under 16 years of age.

Off-label medication can be administered or delegated with an appropriate provider order. The nurse should be familiar with the drug purpose and side-effects in relation to the client that is receiving the medication.

Crushing Tablets

Crushing tablets are usually outside the product licence and nurses should seek advice from a Pharmacist or the prescriber if they are unsure about a tablet and its suitability for crushing, as the process may affect its efficacy. Modified–release tablets must not be crushed as damage to the release-controlling mechanism will result in it negating the modified release aspect and the full dose will be released at once. This could result in toxicity.

Top 100 Most Prescribed Medications in UK Hospitals

Since this chapter is titled 'Drugs and Medicines' lets now look at some medications. According to Public Health England, the following are the most prescribed medications in UK hospitals Table 3.4:

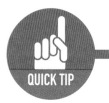

Some medications appear in more than one category.

QUICK TIP

Table 3.4 Top 100 most prescribed medications in UK hospitals.

Category	Information	Medications
Analgesics	These medications help to relieve pain and usually fall into one of several categories: Opioids, non-opioids, non-steroidal anti-inflammatory (NSAID), and 'other'.	Paracetamol Ibuprofen Co-codamol Codeine Tramadol Morphine Diclofenac Aspirin Naproxen Dihydrocodeine Oxycodone Nefopam Gabapentin Fentanyl Katamine Also, long and short acting variants such as Zomorph, oxycontin and MST
Anti-arrhythmics	These medications are used to suppress abnormal rhythms of the heart (cardiac-arrhythmias) such as atrial-fibrillation, atrial flutter, ventricular tachycardia, and ventricular fibrillation.	Fibrillation Bisoprolol Atenolol Digoxin Amiodarone Adenosine Diltiazem
Antibiotics	These medications help the body to fight infection and can be administered orally or intravenously. They usually fall into one of several categories: penicillin's, cephalosporins, aminoglycosides, tetracyclines, macrolides, and fluoroquinolones.	Amoxicillin Flucloxacillin Meropenem Vancomycin Gentamycin Clarithromycin Co-amoxiclav Doxycycline Ceftazidime Piperacillin/ tazobactam (Tazocin) Ciprofloxacin Levofloxacin

(*Continued*)

Table 3.4 (*Continued*)

Category	Information	Medications
		Cephalexin Cefuroxime Clindamycin Trimethoprim Nitrofurantoin
Anti-coagulants	These medications are commonly referred to as 'blood thinners' by members of the general public. These chemical substances true role is to prevent or reduce coagulation of the blood, prolonging the clotting time.	Warfarin Rivaroxaban Apixaban Enoxaparin (Clexane) Funderparinex Heparin
Anti-convulsants	These medications are a diverse group of pharmacological agents used in the treatment of both epileptic and non-epileptic seizures.	Sodium valproate (Epilim) Phenytoin Levetiracetam (Keppra) Gabapentin Clonazepam Diazepam Lorazepam Carbamazepine
Anti-depressants	These medications are used in the treatment of depressive disorders and usually fall into one of the following categories: selective serotonin reuptake inhibitors (SSRis), serotonin-noradrenalin reuptake inhibitors (SNRis), noradrenalin and specific serotonergic antidepressants (NASSA's), and tricyclic antidepressants (TCAs)	Citalopram Fluoxetrine Amitriptyline Sertraline Venlafaxine Mirtazapine Trazodone
Anti-emetics	These medications are used to treat vomiting and nausea and are typically used to treat motion sickness and the side effects of opioid analgesics, general anaesthetics, and chemotherapy directed against cancer.	Cyclizine Ondansertron Metoclopramide Prochlorperazine Levomepromazine

Category	Information	Medications
Anti-hypertensives	These medications are used to treat hypertension and usually fall into one of several categories: angiotensin converting enzyme (ACE) inhibitors, calcium channel blockers (CCBs), angiotensin receptor blockers (ARBs), and beta-blockers. Also see Diuretics.	Ramipril Doxazosin Candesartan Losartan Lisinopril Atenolol Bisoprolol Amiodipine Diltiazem Nifedipine
Anti-hyperglycaemics	These medications are used in the treatments of raised blood sugars, typically in diabetic patients.	Metformin Insulin Gliclazide
Bronchodilators	These medications are used to help make breathing easier by relaxing the muscles of the lungs and widening the bronchi.	Salbutamol Ipratropium Tiotropium Theophylline
Diuretics	These medications increase the production of urine and usually fall into one of several categories: loop diuretics, potassium-sparing diuretics, and thiazides.	Furosemide Bumetanide Spironolactone Bendroflumethiazide Indapamide Amiloride
Intravenous fluids (IVs)	These medications usually fall into one or two categories: Colloid and Crystalloid and can include supplements such as potassium and magnesium.	Normal saline Plasmalyte Hartmann's solution Geloplasma/plasmalyte Glucose
Sedatives	These medications are used for a calming effect. They can be used to promote sleep, ease withdrawal symptoms or reduce agitation and irritability.	Zopiclone Haloperidol Lorazepam Midazolam Diazepam Chlordiazepoxide Temazepam Phenobarbital

(*Continued*)

Table 3.4 (*Continued*)

Category	Information	Medications
Statins or lipid-lowering medications	These are a group of medications used to lower the level of low density lipoprotein (LDL) cholesterol in the blood. They are usually prescribed to help reduce the risk of stroke, coronary heart disease, heart attacks, and angina.	Simvastatin Atorvastatin Pravastatins
Supplements	These medications generally include hormones, vitamins, minerals, fibre, fatty acids or amino acids, and other substances.	Levothyroxine Adcal/calcichew Ferrous fumarate Ferrous sulphate Multivitamins Thiamine Cholecalciferol Quinine Folic acid Sandoz-k Sandoz-phosphate Slow sodium Alendronic acid
Laxatives	These medications are used to treat either acute or chronic constipation and usually fall into one of the following categories: bulk-forming, osmotic, stimulant, or stool softening.	Lactulose Senna Movicol Sodium docusate Bisacodyl Phosphate enema Microlax enema Glycerine suppositories
Proton pump inhibitors (PPis)	These medications are a group of drugs whose main action is to reduce gastric-acid production.	Omeprazole Lansoprazole Esomeprazole Ranitidine (H2 receptor-blocker) Peptac

Source: Public Health England

We will be looking at a handful of these drugs in more detail in Chapter 15.

TEST YOUR KNOWLEDGE

1 What does POM mean?
2 What is a non-proprietary drug name?
3 What is a proprietary drug name?
4 What is a cold chain? Tip: nothing to do with necklaces!
5 The Medicines Act was first introduced when?
6 Give four examples of oral liquid medication formats.
7 In the hospital setting, when checking the prescription chart, the pharmacist will check to see that only approved abbreviations have been used on the chart. We have looked at abbreviations previously. What do the following ones mean?

PO	PR	BD
mg	mL	TDS
IM	NJ	QDS
g	TOP	OM
IV	PV	ON
kg	SL	NG
SC	NEB	PEG
l	OD	

8 Name five anti-emetic drugs.
9 What is the category of drugs used to increase the production of urine?
10 What are Proton Pump Inhibitors?

KEY POINTS

- The categories of medicines.
- Following directions on medication labels and their meanings.
- The differences between non-proprietary names and proprietary names.
- An overview of systemic and topical medications.
- Legislation and Standards around medicines management.
- Looking at the 100 most prescribed medications in UK hospitals.

WEB RESOURCES

RCN: www.rcn.org.uk

Royal Pharmaceutical Society: www.rpharms.com

BNF Adults: www.bnf.nice.org.uk

BNF Children: www.bnfc.nice.org.uk

Public Health England: www.gov.uk/government/
organisation/public-health-england
www.oplc.nh.gov/nursing/documents/off-label-medication

Medicines and Healthcare Products Regulatory Agency:
https://www.mhra.gov.uk

National Patient Safety Agency: www.npsa.nhs.uk

Medications: www.nursingnotes.co.uk/resources/
the-100-most-common-medications
www.medicines.org

Electronic Medicines Compendium: www.medicines.org.uk

Nursing Associates Standards: www.
instituteforapprenticeships.org/apprenticeship-standards/
nursing-associate-nmc-2018/

Chapter 4

CALCULATIONS FOR WORKING OUT DOSAGES

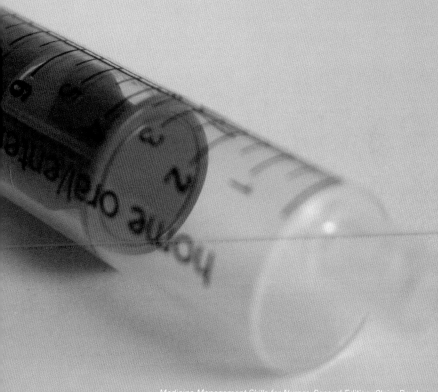

Medicine Management Skills for Nurses, Second Edition. Claire Boyd.
© 2022 John Wiley & Sons Ltd. Published 2022 by John Wiley & Sons Ltd.

LEARNING OUTCOMES

By the end of this chapter you will have an understanding of the theory and practice for working out medication dosages.

Drug administration requires a good grasp of maths and it can really be much simpler that you may have imagined! For example, multiplying and dividing decimals are easy, once you know you just need to bounce the decimal point.

To multiply by	Move the decimal point
10	1 place right
100	2 places right
1000	3 places right

EXAMPLES: 0.798 x 10 = 7.98
0.798 x 100 = 79.8
0.798 x 1000 = 798

NOTE: If the answer is a whole number, the decimal point may be omitted

To divide by	Move the decimal point
10	1 place left
100	2 places left
1000	3 places left

Examples: 0.798/10 = 0.0798
0.798/100 = 0.00798
0.798/1000 = 0.000798

NOTE: A division may be written as a fraction

DRUG DOSAGES FOR TABLETS AND CAPSULES

To work out how many tablets or capsules should be administered to our patient or service user, we must divide what has been prescribed (on the prescription chart) by how the drug has been formatted (how it comes). This is the formula we use:

$$\text{Number of tablets or capsules required} = \frac{\text{what you want}}{\text{what you've got}}$$

Let me show you an example. . .

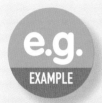

EXAMPLE

You pick up a prescription chart and see that the patient has been prescribed 225 mg of a drug. This is the 'what you want' part of the formula.

There are two tablets in a blister pack in the stock cupboard. This is 'what you've got' part of the formula. Each tablet is equal to 150 mg of the drug. Visualise yourself getting the drug out of the cupboard and popping the pills into a medicine pot.

But you know that two of these tablets will be too much; that is more than what the prescription is asking for. So, you put the figures into the formula and, if using a calculator, input: 225 mg (what you want) divided by 150 mg (what you've got) = 1.5 = 1½ tablets. Therefore, one of these tablets needs to be split in half.

You can only cut tablets in half if they are scored, and never into quarters. Some tablets have an enteric coating or are modified release and cannot be halved (see Chapter 5). Capsules cannot be halved.

GLOSSARY

Enteric coating

Describes drugs that are coated with a substance that enables them to pass through the stomach and the intestine unchanged.

NOTE: it is important when using a formula that all the metric units are the same. For example: if the amount of drug under 'what you want' is in milligrammes then the amount under 'what you've got' has also got to be in milligrammes and not micrograms or grams, etc.

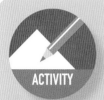

Activity 4.1

How many tablets are required?

1   Prescribed: 225 mg ranitidine; stock strength: 150 mg tablets
2   Prescribed: 750 mg penicillin; stock strength: 250 mg tablets
3   Prescribed: 15 mg codeine phosphate; stock strength: 30 mg tablets
4   Prescribed 150 mg soluble aspirin; stock strength: 300 mg tablets
5   Prescribed: 25 mg captopril; stock strength: 50 mg tablets
6   Prescribed: 125 µg of digoxin; stock strength: 0.25 mg

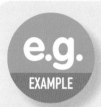

Let me show you an example:

To convert 3500 mg into g = 3500 /1000 = 3.5 g

To convert 2.5 l into ml = 2.5 × 1000 = 2500 ml

DRUG DOSAGES FOR INJECTION (AND ANY LIQUID MEDICATION)

This is the formula we use for any liquid doses, which may be elixirs, linctuses, syrups, or mixtures. It may also be injections. The answer will be in millilitres. This is the formula we use:

$$\text{Volume of drug to be given} = \frac{\text{what you want}}{\text{what you've got}} \times \text{volume}$$

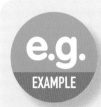

Let me show you an example. . .

A patient is prescribed cortisone 40 mg. The ampoules contain 50 mg in 2 ml. Calculate the volume required for injection.

Using the above formula:

$$\frac{40 \text{ mg}}{50 \text{ mg}} \times 2 \text{ mL} = 1.6 \text{ mL}$$

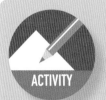

Activity 4.2

Oramorph (liquid) is presented in 100, 300, and 500 ml bottles in strengths of 10 mg/5 ml.

1   Look up and list four possible side effects of opiate medication, and your actions.
2   What is the antidote for an opiate overdose?
3   A patient is prescribed 5 mg of liquid oramorph from a 500 ml bottle. How much do you give?
4   A patient is prescribed 5 mg of liquid oramorph from a 100 ml bottle. How much do you give?
5   A patient is prescribed 7.5 mg of liquid oramorp from a 100 ml bottle. How much do you give?
6   A patient is prescribed 12 mg of liquid oramorp from a 100 ml bottle. How much do you give?

Remember, in this instance, it does not matter what size the bottle, it is the strength that matters in our calculation: 10 mg/5 ml.

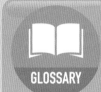

GLOSSARY

Oramorph
Liquid morphine – a strong opioid analgesic

Opiate
A group of drugs derived from opium. Used to relieve pain, suppress coughing, or stimulate vomiting.

INFUSION DEVICES

There are many different types of infusion devices on the market, but Table 4.1 shows us where they fit in with the administration of drugs.

Table 4.1 Infusion devises and administration of drugs.

Infusion device	Used for. . .
Gravity, no pump Equipment required: drip stand, bag of fluid, administration set	These depend on gravity to drive the infusion, counting the drops. Used when administering bags of sodium chloride, dextrose saline, and dextrose infusions. Gravity devices are not generally used for infusions containing potassium or blood (best practise is to use a volumetric pump). Delivers rates in drops per minute.
Volumetric pump Equipment required: used with equipment as for a gravity device	These are used for medium to large flow rates. Used for bags of fluids and blood. Devices usually deliver in rates of millilitres per hour.
Syringe pump (syringe driver) Equipment required: used with a syringe and administration line	Used where small volumes of highly concentrated drugs are required at low flow rates. Used to deliver drugs or infusions in small to medium volumes; calibrated at rates of 0.1–99 ml/h. Often used to deliver heparin and insulin which can be rapidly adjusted depending on patient requirements, and in critical areas drugs such as adrenaline and dobutamine, etc.
Patient-controlled analgesia (PCA) pump Equipment required: used with equipment as for a syringe pump, with a push button or similar device used to deliver the medication on demand	These pumps deliver analgesia to patients, which they administer themselves, according to individual need.
Pump for ambulatory use (syringe driver) Equipment required: used with equipment as for a PCA pump	These small devices can be carried around by patients and are miniature, battery-driven versions of syringe pumps. They usually deliver analgesia, heparin, insulin or cytotoxic drugs. Some devices deliver millilitres per hour whereas other devices deliver millilitres per day.

SYRINGE DRIVERS

A syringe driver is shown in Figure 4.1. This is the formula we use when working out rates for syringe drivers. It is used for setting infusion pump rates in millilitres per hour.

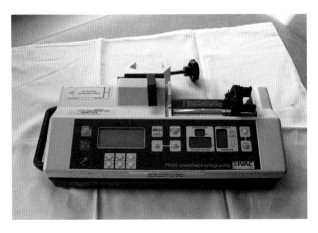

Figure 4.1 A syringe driver.

$$\text{Infusion rate} = \frac{\text{amount of fluid (mL)}}{\text{infustion time (hours)}}$$

Let me show you an example. . .

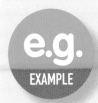

EXAMPLE

25 000 units of heparin have been added to a syringe with sodium chloride 0.9% to make a total amount of 48 ml. This is to be administered over 24 hours. At what rate is the syringe driver to be set?

Using the formula above

$$\frac{48 \text{ mL}}{24 \text{ hours}} = 2 \text{ mL/hour}$$

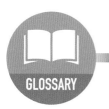

Diamorphine

(also known as heroin). A white crystalline powder derived from morphine. It is a very powerful narcotic analgesic.

GLOSSARY

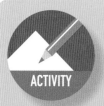

ACTIVITY

Activity 4.3

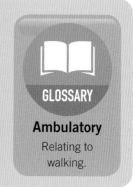

GLOSSARY

Ambulatory
Relating to walking.

Diamorphine has been made up to a total solution of 20 ml in a syringe. It is to be given over 24 hours using a syringe driver. What is the rate in millilitres per hour?

AMBULATORY SYRINGE DRIVERS

Ambulatory syringe drivers are designed for a specific size and make of syringe and can be adjusted to deliver a specific number of millilitres per hour. Others, less commonly used for intravenous drugs, measure *millimetres* (mm) per hour and so the size of the syringe is vitally important to the calculation.

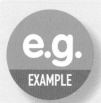

EXAMPLE

Let me show you an example. . .

A prescription for diamorphine 20 mg and cyclizine 50 mg is to be given over 24 hours. The syringe driver, which holds a 10 ml syringe, is set to deliver 2 mm/h. The length of 8 ml in the syringe is measured up as 48 mm.

Diamorphine is available in powder form in 10 mg ampoules. Cyclizine is available in ampoules containing 50 mg/2 ml. How is the solution made up?

Step 1: calculate the total solution required to be delivered at 2 mm/h:

$$2 \text{ mm/hour} \times 24 \text{ hours} = 48 \text{ mm}$$
$$48 \text{ mm} = 8 \text{ mL}$$

Step 2: calculate the volume of water for injection required to dilute the diamorphine:

$$\text{Cyclizine 50 mg} = 2 \text{ mL} \left(50 \text{ mg/2 mL}\right)$$
$$8 \text{ mL} - 2 \text{ mL} = 6 \text{ mL} \left(8 \text{ mL} = 48 \text{ mm}\right)$$
Dilute the 20 mg diamorphine with 6 mL of water.

Therefore in the syringe is 8 ml = 48 mm:

2 mL of this is cyclizine
6 mL of this is diamorphine

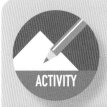

Activity 4.4

ACTIVITY

The prescription is diamorphine 30 mg, cyclizine 50 mg/1 ml to be administered over 24 hours using a syringe driver that holds a 10 ml syringe. Cyclizine comes in 50 mg/ml vials.

1   How much water for injection is required to make up an 8 ml syringe?
2   If every 10 mg of diamorphine is to be diluted with 1 ml of sterile water, how much water is required to make the 8 ml syringe?
3   What rate should the syringe driver be set at to deliver the 8 ml over 24 hours?

GRAVITY-FEED DRIP RATES (DROPS PER MINUTE)

This is the formula we use to administer bags of fluid and blood when we do not have a pump (see a gravity-feed drip in Figure 4.2). It depends on what liquid we are infusing as to the administration set we use:

$$\text{Rate} = \frac{\text{volume}}{\text{time in hours}} \times \frac{\text{drops per millilitre}}{\text{minutes per hour}}$$

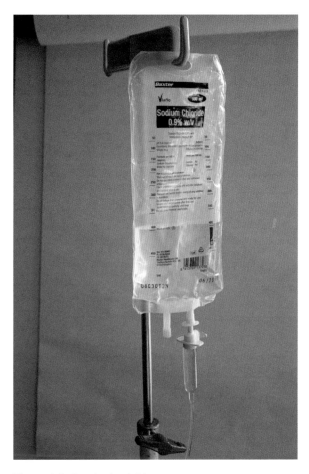

Figure 4.2 Gravity-feed drip.

Let's break the formula up into parts to make sense of it: the volume is the amount that has been prescribed, such as 1 l of sodium chloride 0.9%. The time in hours is also what has been prescribed by the medic, say 'to be given over eight hours'.

The minutes per hour is always going to 60, as there are only 60 minutes in an hour! The number of drops per millilitre depends on the type of fluid being infused and the type of giving set (or administration set) in use. In general, check the infusion set's packaging for the flow rate.

Blood administration or standard giving set:

Blood and 'thick' fluids = 15 drops/ml
Clear fluids = 20 drops/ml

Microdrip or paediatric giving set, sometimes referred to as a microdrop burette:

Clear fluids = 60 drops/ml

Putting this all together, we work this out as:

Volume amount divided by time in hours multiplied by drops/ml (depending on the infusate) divided by minutes per hour (always 60)

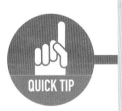

QUICK TIP

Best practice is to deliver blood and blood products through a volumetric pump. Some community settings may administer blood via gravity, so it is important for you to know how to work out the drip rate.

Giving an infusion containing potassium via gravity can also be dangerous. Check your institution's IV policy on potassium delivery.

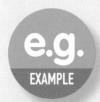

Let me show you an example. . .

A patient is to receive 1 l of 5% glucose in eight hours. Calculate the rate in drops per minute, using a standard giving set (20 drops/ml).

Using the above formula:

$$\frac{1000 \text{ mL}}{8 \text{ hours}} \times \frac{20 \text{ drops/mL}}{60 \text{ minutes}} = 41.6$$

Answer = 42 drops per minute (rounding to the nearest drop)

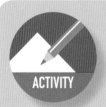

Activity 4.5

50 ml of Hartmann's solution is to be given to a child over one hour. Calculate the rate in drops per minute using a paediatric/microdrip giving set.

DURATION OF INFUSION

When we need to work out how long our infusion has left to run through, this is the formula we use:

Duration of Infusion

$$\frac{\text{Volume}}{\begin{array}{c}\text{Rate of infusion}\\\text{(Drops per minute)}\end{array}} \times \frac{\text{Drops per millilitre}}{60 \text{ Minutes}}$$

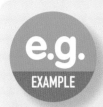

Let me show you an example. . .

600 ml of fluid is dripping at 20 drops per minute. The intravenous (IV) set delivers 15 drops/ml. How long will the infusion take?

$$\frac{600 \text{ mL}}{20 \text{ drops per minute}} \times \frac{15 \text{ drops/mL}}{60 \text{ minutes}} = 7\frac{1}{2} \text{ hours}$$

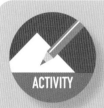

Activity 4.6

Half a litre of fluid is being given at 25 drops per minute, 15 drops/ml. How long will the infusion take?

DRUGS ACCORDING TO BODY WEIGHT

When we need to titrate drugs according to body weight, this is the formula we use:

$$\text{Correct dosage per day} = \frac{\text{weight}(\text{kg})}{\times \text{dose per kg}}$$

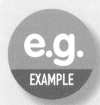

Let me show you an example. . .

A patient is prescribed streptomycin 30 mg per kg per day in three doses. The patient weighs 48 kg. Calculate the quantity of drug required for each dose.

$$48 \text{ kg} \times 30 \text{ mg/kg} = 1440 \text{ mg/day}$$

$$\frac{1440 \text{ mg/day}}{3} = 480 \text{ mg per dose}$$

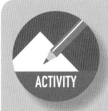

Activity 4.7

Erythromycin 40 mg per kg per day is prescribed in four doses to a 12 kg child. Work out the amount in a single dose.

SETTING PUMPS TO RUN AT MILLILITRES PER HOUR

Some pumps are set to deliver the dose in millilitres per hour.

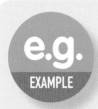

Let me show you an example. . .

If we have 750 ml of Hartmann's solution to administer over six hours we can input these figures into the machine:

$$\frac{750 \text{ mL}}{6 \text{ hours}} = 125 \text{ mL/hour}$$

We can reverse-check this by seeing that $125 \times 6 = 750$ ml.

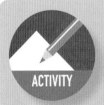

Activity 4.8

5000 units of heparin has been made up to a total amount of 48 ml with sodium chloride 0.9%. This is to be given over 16 hours using a pump. Input these figures into the infusion device, and state the number of millilitres per hour to be delivered.

TEST YOUR KNOWLEDGE

1   Prescribed: 15 mg nortriptyline; stock strength: 10 mg. How many tablets are required?
2   Cough syrup is presented as 10 mg/ml. How many millilitres are required for a prescribed dose of 15 mg?
3   A patient has been prescribed one unit of blood (350 ml) to run over three hours. What is the drip rate in drops per minute?

4   An infusion is dripping at 20 drops per minute. The IV administration set delivers 20 drops per ml. How long will the infusion take? 700 ml has already been delivered from the 1 l bag of fluid.

5   A patient weighs 90 kg and has been prescribed 40 mg per kg per day of a drug. Calculate the dose required.

6   A patient is to receive 48 ml of a drug over 12 hours. What is the rate in millilitres per hour?

KEY POINTS

- How to calculate dosages for oral (including liquid) and injectable drug dosages.
- Looking at infusion devices used to administer medications.
- How to calculate infusion pump rates.
- How to calculate gravity drip rates (in drops per minute) and the duration of these infusions.
- How to calculate drugs according to body weight

WEB RESOURCES

Maths: www.testandcalc.com/quiz/index.asp
Maths is Fun: www.mathisfun.com/tables.html
British National Formulary: www.bnf.nice.org.uk

Chapter 5
. . . .
ORAL DRUG ADMINISTRATION

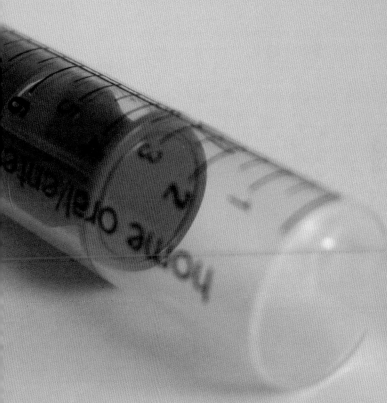

Medicine Management Skills for Nurses, Second Edition. Claire Boyd.
© 2022 John Wiley & Sons Ltd. Published 2022 by John Wiley & Sons Ltd.

Let's start at the very beginning – the legal documents we use for administering medications.

THE PRESCRIPTION CHART

Now let's look at the prescription chart (see Appendix 2), which is used in the hospital setting. This is a typical prescription chart, but they do vary slightly from Trust to Trust. On the front page you will notice that it has room to put all our patient's details, such as name, date of birth, unit number, weight, and any allergies or sensitivities they may have. All these details must be completed. We also have a section for the pharmacy to write any instructions for us to see. The front section also contains the oxygen therapy prescription. Did you know that oxygen is a prescribed drug? Without a prescription it can only be given in an emergency situation.

There is also a section for 'once only and premedication drugs': this is usually for one-off prescriptions, perhaps for someone going to surgery where the medic prescribes something like 10 mg diazepam, orally.

On the front page of the chart, we can see that there is a section for drug allergies or sensitivities but also includes *anything* to which the patient considers themselves sensitive or allergic.

Certain foodstuffs are linked to latex proteins, so if a patient informs us that they are allergic to kiwi fruit, bananas, or avocado, they are probably allergic to latex because these food items have the same protein chains as latex. The patient must then be considered as latex sensitive. Any equipment used with this patient must be latex-free. This is why it is vital that a good, robust admission procedure is performed on each patient so that their medical history is fully known. Details can then be written on the prescription chart to alert colleagues; this goes on the front of the chart where it states Drug allergies/sensitivities. In this case you would write 'allergic to bananas'.

On the second page of the prescription chart (see the second page of Appendix 2) the regular prescriptions are written in and our patient's details are replicated. If our patient requires analgesia for 'breakthrough' pain or night sedation, this will be written in the 'as required' section. Antibiotics must have a Stop date documented, such as five days for oral antibiotics.

Next we have the administration record (see the third page of Appendix 2), where the nurse or nurses need to sign their initials. Nursing Associates, Assistant Practitioners, and Operating Department Practitioners who have been trained to administer drugs also need to sign here. We also document the time that a medication is given.

Never sign for medication and leave it on the cabinet for the patient 'to take later'. *You are signing to say you have seen the drugs being swallowed.* Anyone can pick up drugs that have been left around the ward. Also, it is important that timed drugs are taken at the correct time. A patient left to his or her own devices might not take a dose that has been left for three or four hours, and if the medication is to be given every four hours the result could be an overdose.

You will notice that we have code numbers for the **omission of medications**:

1 allergic reaction,
2 patient fasting,
3 omitted for clinical reasons (the reason must be documented on the back page of the chart),
4 patient refused,
5 patient unavailable,
6 drug unavailable.

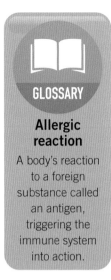

Patients classified as Nil by mouth should still have their prescribed oral medications administered to them at the prescribed time unless this has specifically been advised against, and documented otherwise. It is the responsibility of the prescriber to provide clear written instructions to nursing staff concerning the omission of prescribed doses.

On the final page of the prescription chart (see the fourth page of Appendix 2) we write the reasons for not giving a prescribed medication. For instance, a patient complaining of diarrhoea we would omit their prescribed senna and lactulose. We would need to record why we did not give the drug.

Also, we would not wake a patient for night sedation if they were already asleep. But we would need to document the reason why this medication was omitted, otherwise it would seem as though we had either forgotten to give the drug or forgotten to document that we had given the drug. It is classed as neglect if a drug has been omitted for no good reason, and an accident/incident form will need to be completed.

Specialist wound care prescriptions are recorded here, as are the medications that the patient needs to take home with them. Many institutions call this the TTA, which is short for the patient 'to take away', or TTO, short for 'tablets to take out'.

Electronic Prescription Charts – Bar-Coding

Many hospitals now have a system of computer prescriptions using a hand-held device. The nurse swipes their own authorisation identity badge and the patient's wristband, which contains a chip that stores the patient's prescription with all the correct dosages already calculated. This system is used in some parts of the USA and is said to prevent medication errors.

In a drive to become 'paperless' prescription charts may become a thing of the past, with us all using computer devices to access patient drug charts. But what if we rely on a computer and the computer makes a mistake?

Community Medication Administration Sheet (MAR)

The MAR sheet is the medication document used in the community (Service Users own home or in the care home environment). Just like the hospital prescription form, these sheets can vary from care environment to care environment and can be a paper copy or electronic. In some areas they are known as Medication Administration Records and Request form (MARR). The MARR is the place to record:

- Ordering of medicines
- Receipt of medicines
- Dosing instructions
- Emergency supplies and interims
- Unwanted/discontinued medications
- Any medications not prescribed by the General Practitioner (GP)
- Controlled drugs

Care Home Homely Remedy

These are medicines that may normally be bought by an individual without calling a GP. This is a locally agreed list and include such medicines such as Strepsils and cough syrup – in fact the sort of thing we have in our own medicine cabinets. In the care home situation, the GP should be informed about any homely remedy taken by the Service User/Resident to check that it will not cause any harm with any prescribed drugs they may be taking.

Now let's look at the world of the oral route.

ORAL ROUTES

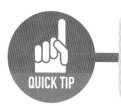

QUICK TIP

Do not interfere with time-release medication or medication with an enteric coating.

Inform the patient that they will need to swallow this medication whole and not to chew.

Modified-Release Medications

Such tablets and capsules have special coatings and release the drug over time. These drugs are prescribed on the prescription chart as m/r or retard (meaning modified-release) which can be slow or continuous. An example of this is MST Continuous (morphine sulphate tablets), which are designed to work continuously for 12 hours.

Medications with an Enteric Coating

These drugs have a coating to protect the stomach on their way into the system. You will see on the prescription chart EN or Enteric coated (EC) at the end of the drug name. An example of this is Aspirin EC.

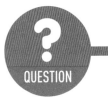

QUESTION

Question 5.1   If your were asked to administer medications via the sublingual route or the buccal route, where would you place this medication?

The sublingual mucosa has a rich blood supply through which drugs can be absorbed rapidly into the systemic circulation. The most common example of a drug administered via this route is glyceryl trinitrate, which is used to treat acute angina.

How to Calculate Oral Drug Dosages

When working out how many tablets or capsules to administer for drug administration, some calculations can be quite simple.

For example, paracetamol is presented as 500 mg per tablet. If a patient requires (is prescribed) 1000 mg we can see that two tablets are required (500 + 500 = 1000 mg). This is known as the calculations 'bundles' approach.

$$\text{Number of tablets or capsules required} = \frac{\text{what you want}}{\text{what you've got}}$$

This means what you want *divided* by what you've got.

The formula approach comes into its own when we have more complicated calculations to work out. However, an understanding of the whys and wherefores of the problem must first be established; that is, what are we doing and why? In addition, we should always be thinking around the box: does the answer look right? This means we should have made a rough 'guesstimate' of the answer.

NOTE: 'what you want' is what has been prescribed and we divide this by how the medication is presented in its blister pack or bottle, which is the 'what you've got' part.

SOLID ORAL MEDICINES

Using a Tablet Cutter

Figures 5.1a,b shows a tablet cutter that can also crush drugs. You should only cut tablets in half if they are scored, and never into quarters. Some tablets have an enteric coating or are modified release and cannot be halved. Capsules cannot be halved.

(a)   (b)

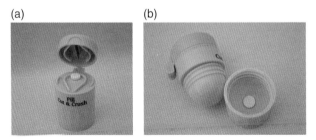

Figure 5.1 (a) Cutting and (b) crushing a tablet.

You must remember to clean a tablet cutter after using it.

Crushing of Solid Oral Medicines

If a patient is unable to swallow solid oral medications, the pharmacy should be contacted about the availability of an alternative liquid formulation of the drug. This is due to the fact that not all drugs *can* be crushed.

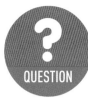

Question 5.2   Why should you never use a mortar and pestle to crush drugs in the clinical area?

Swallowing Difficulties

Some patients may experience difficulties with swallowing, known as dysphagia. When administering medications, we need to be vigilant, observing for any signs and symptoms that our patient or service user is experiencing any difficulties. We must look for:

- Pain while chewing,
- Pain while swallowing,
- Complaining of a dry mouth,
- Difficulty in controlling food and/or liquids in the mouth,
- Hoarse or wet voice,
- Coughing or choking before, during or after swallowing,
- Regurgitation of undigested food,
- Recurrent chest infections,
- Unexplained weight loss.

Some medications may make the active process of swallowing more problematic in those experiencing dysphagia, as certain drugs are known to cause a dry mouth (see Table 5.1).

Table 5.1 Drugs that may be difficult to swallow.

Type of drug	Example
Tricyclic antidepressants	Amitriptyline
Other types of antidepressants	Fluoxetine
Antihistamines	Chlorphenamine
Antimuscarinic drugs	Hyoscine
Certain antipsychotics	Haloperidol
Certain beta-blockers	Carvedilol
Certain diuretics	Triamterene

LIQUID MEDICATIONS

Not all oral medications come as tablets or capsules. Oral medication may also be presented in a liquid format (see Table 5.2), such as cough syrups, elixirs, and linctuses.

Table 5.2 Liquid medications.

Type of liquid medication	Characteristics
Elixir	Clear or flavoured oral liquid containing one or more active ingredients.
Linctus	Viscous oral liquid containing one or more active ingredients; commonly used as cough medications.
Syrup	Does not contain any active ingredients.
Mixture	Flavoured solutions or suspension of drug, used when a patient has difficulty swallowing or a drug is not available in tablet format. Must be shaken well before administration to mix the contents thoroughly.

Having a liquid form means that our medication will need to be worked out in millilitres. This is the formula that we use:

$$\text{Volume of drug to be given} = \frac{\text{what you want}}{\text{what you've got}} \times \text{volume}$$

Let me show you an example: a child has been prescribed 6 mg of cough mixture. The medication and stock ampoules contain 10 mg/ml. What I want = 6 mg, what I've got = 10 mg and what it comes in (volume) = 1 ml:

6 mg divided by 10 mg multiplied by 1 ml = 0.6 ml. So, I draw up 0.6 ml knowing that there is 6 mg of the drug in my syringe.

Looking at the whole picture, I know this looks about right as my answer should indeed be *under* the 1 ml mark, as this is how much liquid holds 10 mg of the drug, and I want less than this.

I can use a measuring pot (Figure 5.2) to pour my liquid medication, or I can use an oral syringe (Figure 5.3). When using a measuring pot, the eye must be level with the lower line of the meniscus.

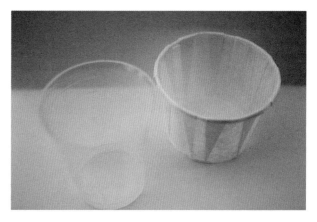

Figure 5.2 A plastic measuring pot and a wax tablet pot.

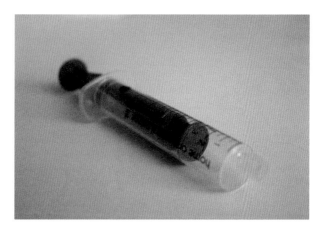

Figure 5.3 An oral syringe.

What's A Meniscus?

The surface tension of a liquid causes it to have a curved surface as the edges of the liquid climb up the sides of the container. This is called the meniscus (see Figure 6.6). To accurately measure the liquid in a medicine pot or syringe, you read the bottom of the curve where it is at its lowest, in the middle (bottom of the meniscus), not the top of the curve (top of the meniscus).

SERVICE USERS

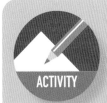

Activity 5.1

Let's imagine you are qualified and working in the community, going into service users' homes. How do you answer the following questions?

1 What would you do if a service user refuses to take their medication?
2 How do you measure liquid preparations when pouring them?
3 Is it acceptable to crush tablets or open capsules and sprinkle the contents on food?
4 Why is it important to store liquids correctly as directed on the packaging, e.g. in the fridge or in brown bottles?
5 What is a 'dosette box'?
6 What would you do if a service user has taken an over-the-counter medication containing paracetamol, and who is now due paracetamol from the dosette box?
7 What would you do if you drop or spoil medication you are about to administer?
8 Why is it important to consider 'time of administration' when administering medications?
9 Why should some liquid medications be shaken prior to administering?
10 You have just given a new medication to a service user, who now becomes unwell. What do you do?
11 What is a use-by date?
12 How should tablets/capsules be administered to service users? Is it acceptable to give them from your clean hands?
13 What would you do if you give the service user the wrong drug?

SELF-ADMINISTRATION OF DRUGS

Adult patients who have been screened by the multi-disciplinary team may be permitted to self-medicate their medication while in hospital. The rationale for self-medication is to be proactive in improving compliance and concordance. In other words, there will be:

- Increased patient satisfaction,
- Better preparation for discharge,
- Effective use of medication following discharge.

Of course, some patients will be unable to participate in this scheme. Patient exclusion criteria will vary between hospital trusts, but may include:

- Those patients thought to be at risk of deliberate overdose;
- Those patients being discharged to nursing homes;
- Patients with unstable mental health conditions (unless only on antidepressants);
- Controlled drugs: patients must not self-administer these;
- Those too ill or confused to be ultimately discharged to live alone;
- Those patients on compliance devices filled by a community pharmacist (e.g. dosette boxes);
- If patients are identified as having difficulty in opening bottles or reading labels then this should be brought to the attention of the pharmacist so that the problems can be addressed.

Many areas have a staged self-medication schedule, whereby patients are assessed as to the level of self-medication that is suitable. They can then be moved up or down these levels as required. This may be:

Level 1   Medicines are locked in a medication locker. Nurse administers the medication, giving a full explanation.

Level 2   As for level 1 except that the patient will be encouraged to ask the nursing staff to open the cabinet.

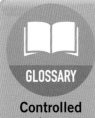

GLOSSARY

Controlled drugs

Drugs that are controlled under the Misuse of Drugs legislation; for example, morphine, pethidine, and methadone (also see Chapter 3).

Level 3   Medicines are locked in the medication locker. The key is kept with the patient. The patient administers their medicines without direct supervision. The nurse checks compliance and suitability verbally.

The prescription chart should be highlighted to indicate which items are being self-medicated.

Individuals at home and self-administering in the hospital may have difficulty opening their medication due to a child-resistant screw top (such as a clic loc cap) having been placed onto the medication bottle. It may be necessary to ask the Pharmacist to supply the medication in a screw top only cap.

DID YOU KNOW?

I went to the chemist to pick up a prescription. The Pharmacist said that when taking the medication, I may experience irritability and pain in my hand and wrist. And that's just from trying to get the cap off! LOL

CONTROLLED DRUGS

Controlled drugs are stored and locked away in a controlled drug cupboard. The keys for this cupboard should be kept separate from other ward keys.

Controlled drugs are counted in when new supplies arrive and counted out when required by a patient's prescription chart. These are checked by two health-care professionals and are signed out in the controlled drug book, when administering to patients. Community settings may not have the luxury of a second checker as one may not be available, so extra vigilance will be required.

Regular checks of the controlled drugs are made, to monitor for any discrepancies.

CHECKING MEDICATIONS FOR CHILDREN

Children are often defined within the healthcare environment as any patient under the age of 12 years; you will need to check your own area. When paediatric drug doses are calculated according to the weight of the child it is essential that this is recorded in kilogrammes on the prescription chart, and this weight must be checked at regular, agreed, intervals. This is the formula we use to titrate medications according to body weight:

$$\text{Weight}\,(\text{kg}) \times \text{dose}$$

For example, if we had a small baby weighing 2 kg and a drug was prescribed as 1.5 mg/kg, we would use the formula above, which works out as $2 \times 1.5 = 3$ mg of the drug either per day or per hour, according to the prescription.

This formula is used a lot in paediatrics and neonatal care, critical care, and in care of the elderly.

It is also a statutory requirement that date of birth is recorded on the prescription.

All drugs administered to children need to be second-checked. Some areas allow this to be a parent/guardian in exceptional circumstances, so you will need to check this in your own clinical environment.

Many areas do not ask for the following drugs to be second-checked, but again you will need to find out what is acceptable protocol in your area:

- paracetamol,
- ibuprofen,
- vitamin supplements,
- nystatin suspension and cream,
- salbutamol nebules,
- eardrops,
- dietary supplements,
- laxatives, aperients, and enemata,
- immunisations.

Children Who Refuse Their Medication

When administering medication to children, we should, as the administrator, take into account their age and level of understanding. Where it is considered that a child recognises the implications of refusing medication, medical staff are informed and the incident recorded in the medical notes. If the child is considered incapable of recognising the implications of refusing medication, provided parental consent is given, the medication should be administered.

Administration to Children by a Parent/ Guardian

Parents or guardians may administer the prescribed medicine to their child, but it is the nurse who takes overall responsibility for ensuring that the medication has been given.

ADMINISTRATION

Procedure for Oral Drug Administration

1   Wash your hands.
2   Check the prescription chart: is the medication now due, has it already been administered, is the prescription clear and legible, does the patient have any allergies or sensitivities and are there any special instructions, such as 'take with food'? Do not break tablets unless they are scored; if appropriate, a tablet cutter must be used.
3   Check:
    drug,
    dose,
    date and time of administration,
    route and method of administration,
    validity of prescription,
    signature of prescribing practitioner.
4   Select the medication and check the expiry date.
5   Do not touch the medication: empty the drugs into a container using the non-touch technique.

6   Take the medication and prescription chart to the patient. Check the patient's identity band and ask them to state their name and date of birth (if able). Discuss with patient the medication being administered and gain their informed consent.

7   Offer a glass of water, and suggest that the patient takes a sip first.

8   Observe the patient taking the medication.

9   Record the dose given, and time and date. Sign the chart.

10   Monitor the patient for any possible side effects or adverse reactions.

Procedure for Administering Medication to Children and Babies using an Oral Syringe

1   Gently push the oral syringe into the side of the mouth.

2   Slowly push the contents of the syringe out into the child's cheek.

3   Pause to allow the contents to be swallowed.

NOTE: it may be appropriate to sit the child on a parent's or guardian's knee during this procedure in order to soothe the child and facilitate co-operation.

TEST YOUR KNOWLEDGE

Look at the completed page 2 of a prescription chart shown in Figure 5.4, and note the drugs listed. The medications come in the formats given below. How many tablets or capsules do you need to administer?

1   Erythromycin: on hand are 250 mg tablets. What is the dose per day?

2   Aspirin (dispersible tablets): on hand are 75 mg tablets. How is this medication to be given?

3   Propranolol hydrochloride: on hand are 160 mg capsules. What is the dose per day?

6 hourly	06.00 – 12.00 – 18.00 – 24.00	SURNAME (MR/MRS/MISS)	DATE OF BIRTH	UNIT NUMBER
8 hourly	06.00 – 14.00 – 22.00	FIRST NAMES	SEX	CONSULTANT
12 hourly	09.00 – 21.00	ADDRESS		

REGULAR PRESCRIPTIONS

	Date	Drug (approved name – BLOCK CAPITALS)	Dose	Route	Times of Administration				Other Directions/ Duration	Doctor's Signature	Date	Pharm
					6	12	18	23				
1	TODAY	ERYTHROMYCIN	500MG	0	√	√	√	√		A Doctor		
2	TODAY	ASPIRIN (DISPERSIBLE)	300MG	0			√		AFTER FOOD	A Doctor		
3	TODAY	PROPRANOLOL	80MG	0		√	√			A Doctor		
4												
5												
6												
7												
8												
9												
10												
11												
12												
13												
14												
15												
16												

AS REQUIRED PRESCRIPTIONS

	Date	Drug (approved name – BLOCK CAPITALS)	Dose	Route	Directions	Maximum Frequency	Doctor's Signature	Date	Pharm
1									
2									
3									
4									
5									
6									
7									
8									
9									
10									

Figure 5.4 Page 2 of a patient's prescription chart, completed by a doctor. Source: Reproduced here with permission from North Bristol NHS Trust and University Hospitals Bristol NHS Foundation Trust.

KEY POINTS

- Looking at the prescription chart document in full.
- The oral route of drug administration and how to work out dosages.
- Factors around patients who self-administer their medications.
- The strict controls around 'controlled drugs'.
- The administration of medications to children.

WEB RESOURCES

Electronic Medicines Compendium: www.emcmedicines.org.uk

BNF for Adults: www.bnf.nice.org.uk

BNF for Children: www.bnfc.nice.org.uk

Chapter 6
· ·
ADMINISTRATION OF INJECTIONS

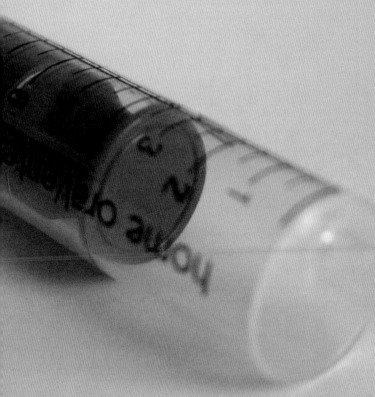

Medicine Management Skills for Nurses, Second Edition. Claire Boyd.
© 2022 John Wiley & Sons Ltd. Published 2022 by John Wiley & Sons Ltd.

LEARNING OUTCOMES

By the end of this chapter you will understand both the theory and practise behind the clinical skill of administering injections. Also vaccine development.

REASONS FOR ADMINISTERING MEDICATION BY INJECTION

Some medications need to be administered by injection, rather than a tablet, oral liquid, or by topical application.

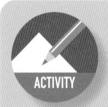

Activity 6.1

Why do some drugs need to be administered via injection? List five possible reasons.

PARENTERAL DRUG ADMINISTRATION

Routes

Parenteral drug administration actually means any non-oral means of drug administration, but now tends to generally refers to the injectable route. The most common routes of parenteral administration you may see are:

- intramuscular (IM),
- subcutaneous (SC),
- intravenous (IV).

Disadvantages of Parental Drug Administration

Although we have looked at the advantages of parental drug administration, there is always a yin to the yang. The disadvantages of this route of administration are:

- It requires trained staff to administer, and sometimes two to check prescriptions, etc.
- It can be more costly that the same medication in another format.
- It can be painful for the patient.
- Aseptic technique is required: this corner must not be cut due to the risk of systemic infection.
- It may require supporting equipment, such as infusion devices. Staff need to be trained to use these devices.

NOTE: IV bolus injections will be discussed in Chapter 11.

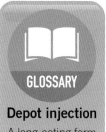

GLOSSARY

Depot injection
A long-acting form of subcutaneous or intramuscular injection.

DEPOT INJECTIONS

Certain types of injectable drug can be injected into the muscle or adipose tissue beneath the skin to allow a deposit or 'depot' of the drug that will be released gradually into the systemic circulation over a period of time. This is often used as a means of administering antipsychotic agents such as flupenthixol in oil, which then needs to be administered just once a month or every three months.

SYRINGES

Syringes (Figure 6.1) are used to inject medications via the intradermal (within the skin), subcutaneous, intramuscular, or intravenous routes. In the neurosciences medics also use a route known as intrathecal, which is within the meninges of the spinal cord.

There are many reasons why we would need to give patients their medication with a syringe and needle via one of these routes. For instance, patients may be unable to swallow, or unable to tolerate medications and fluid via the enteral (oral) route. A medication may also not come in an oral format (such as insulin) if it is destroyed by chemicals in the intestine. An injection of analgesia is more quickly absorbed by the body than a tablet or capsule, which is again a good reason for an injectable format to be chosen. Not all syringes will need to have a needle attached when administering, as there are oral syringes (Figure 6.2), often used in paediatrics to measure and administer oral medications.

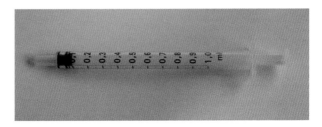

Figure 6.1 A syringe.

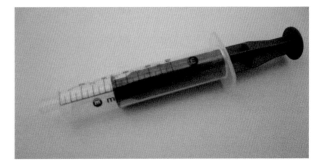

Figure 6.2 An oral syringe.

NOTE: oral syringes are not the same as other syringes.

The Syringe

The syringe is made up of a barrel to contain the liquid that is drawn up, with calibrations marked along the outer surface. A moveable plunger is contained inside the barrel with an end tip. Pulling this plunger back sucks fluid into the barrel and pushing it in, or forward, expels this fluid. Syringes have an end tip, of different varieties and placements, in order for a needle to be attached.

Types of Syringe

Luer-lock These are for secure connections, whereby the needle is screwed onto the syringe (Figure 6.3).

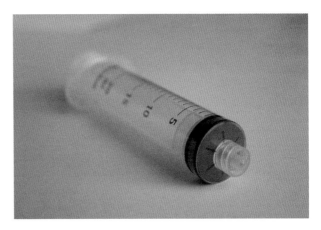

Figure 6.3 A Luer-lock syringe.

Eccentric Luer-slip This is where the nozzle is off-centre to allow closer application to the skin (Figure 6.4).

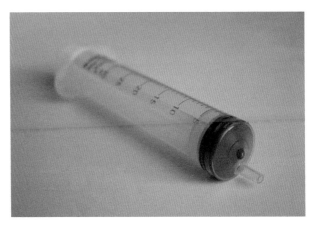

Figure 6.4 An eccentric Luer-slip syringe.

Concentric Luer-slip This is used for all other applications. The nozzle is in the centre (Figure 6.5).

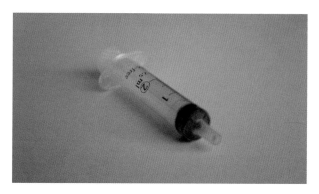

Figure 6.5 A concentric Luer-slip syringe.

Syringes come in various sizes with different calibrations:

1 ml syringes have divisions of 0.01 ml,
2 ml syringes have divisions of 0.1 ml,
5 ml syringes have divisions of 0.2 ml,
10, 20, and 50 ml syringes have 1 ml divisions.

Insulin

Insulin is administered using a special insulin syringe. Insulin is prepared in units per millilitre, in vials that contain 100 units/ml: these are known as multi-dose vials. The standard insulin syringe is calibrated in 2-unit divisions up to 100 units. Patients may require only a small dose (less than 50 units) and so there are also low-dose 0.5 ml syringes available that are graduated in 1-unit divisions up to 50 units.

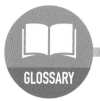

GLOSSARY

Insulin
A protein hormone produced in the pancreas. Important for regulating glucose in the blood.

Heparin

Like insulin, heparin is prescribed in units and drawn up in a 1 ml syringe. It also comes in pre-filled syringes. Heparin is available in single- or multi-dose vials, in various strengths, such as:

1000 units/ml,
5000 units/ml,
25 000 units/ml,
5000 units/5 ml,
25 000 units/5 ml.

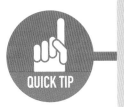

QUICK TIP

You may still see some medics writing units on prescription charts as International Units (IU), meaning International Units. This can be confused with IV for intravenous, so the word units is now preferred.

Don't confuse units with millilitres!

NOTE: a syringe should ideally only be filled to 75% capacity. This is in order for any re-adjustments to be made when drawing up, and is especially important when injecting into muscle, and drawing back to establish that we are not about to inject the medication into a blood vessel. You may have noticed that a 50 ml syringe in fact goes up to 60 ml.

The surface tension of a liquid causes it to produce a curved surface as the edges of the liquid climb up the sides of the container. This is called the meniscus. To accurately measure the liquid in a medicine pot or syringe, you read the bottom of the curve where it is at its lowest, in the middle (bottom of the meniscus), not the top of the curve (top of the meniscus).

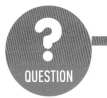

QUESTION

Question 6.1   What is the reading on the meniscus in Figure 6.6?

Practise reading the meniscus levels of medications in syringes and medicine pots: always read the lowest level of the curve, and always at eye level to obtain an accurate reading.

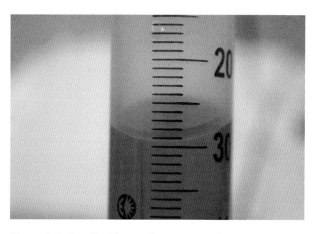

Figure 6.6 Reading the meniscus on a syringe.

Ideally, when drawing up medication from an ampoule or vial, a specialised blunt filter needle should be used, but these may not be readily available. Therefore, it is considered best practice to use a small needle (23 gauge, or 23g) to reduce the possibility of drawing up shards of glass or particles of the rubber from these receptacles. After the medication has been drawn up the needle needs to be replaced with a new, appropriately sized needle, prior to administration.

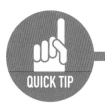

QUICK TIP

The larger the number on a needle, the smaller the needle.

NEEDLES

Needles come in gauge sizes. The three most common needles you may use in practise are:

40 mm $(21$ gauge$)$ = quite large needle
25 mm $(23$ g$)$ = quite small needle
16 mm $(25$ g$)$ = very small needle, often used for subcutaneous injections

The higher the gauge, the finer the bore.

Needles for Injection

Needles consist of a hub and the tip of the needle is bevelled: this is a 'cut out' (Figure 6.7). The bevel is uppermost when injecting for intradermal injections, and downwards for all other injections. IM injections into the buttocks tend to be with either a 21 or 23 g needle. The size of needle depends on the patient's size: 21 g is suitable for most adults and obese adults, whereas 23 g is suitable for very thin adults.

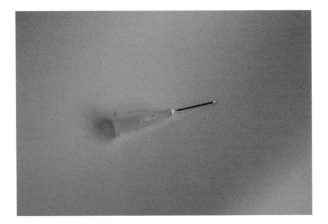

Figure 6.7 A bevelled needle.

For IM injections into the thigh and arm the 23 g is suitable for most adults.

For SC injections the 25 g needle tends to be used.

INJECTIONS

The routes most commonly used for the administration of injections are the subcutaneous (SC; beneath the skin), the intramuscular (IM; into muscle), and the intravenous (IV; into a vein) routes. The buttocks tend to be the most common site for IM injections, but due to the presence of nerves in this region, especially the sciatic nerve, this may give rise to nerve damage. The sites used for IM injections tend to be the deltoid (arm), ventrogluteal, dorsogluteal (both buttock muscles, the upper outer quadrant of the buttock), and vastus lateralis (middle outer aspect of the thigh) muscles. Look up these muscles in an anatomy and physiology textbook. Some are shown in Figure 6.8.

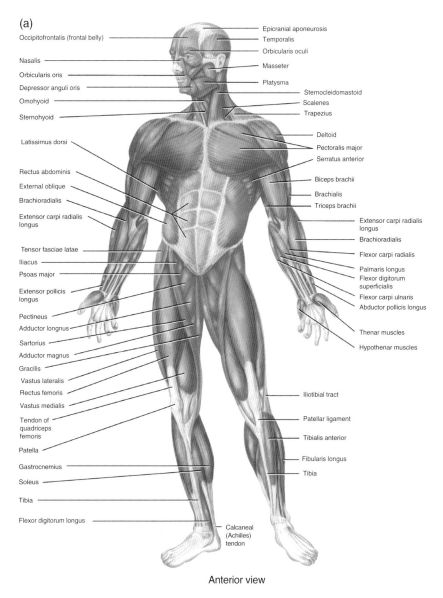

(a)

Occipitofrontalis (frontal belly)

Nasalis

Orbicularis oris

Depressor anguli oris

Omohyoid

Sternohyoid

Latissimus dorsi

Rectus abdominis

External oblique

Brachioradialis

Extensor carpi radialis longus

Tensor fasciae latae

Iliacus

Psoas major

Extensor pollicis longus

Pectineus

Adductor longnus

Sartorius

Adductor magnus

Gracilis

Vastus lateralis

Rectus femoris

Vastus medialis

Tendon of quadriceps femoris

Patella

Gastrocnemius

Soleus

Tibia

Flexor digitorum longus

Epicranial aponeurosis

Temporalis

Orbicularis oculi

Masseter

Platysma

Sternocleidomastoid

Scalenes

Trapezius

Deltoid

Pectoralis major

Serratus anterior

Biceps brachii

Brachialis

Triceps brachii

Extensor carpi radialis longus

Brachioradialis

Flexor carpi radialis

Palmaris longus

Flexor digitorum superficialis

Flexor carpi ulnaris

Abductor pollicis longus

Thenar muscles

Hypothenar muscles

Iliotibial tract

Patellar ligament

Tibialis anterior

Fibularis longus

Tibia

Calcaneal (Achilles) tendon

Anterior view

Figure 6.8 (*Continued*)

(b)

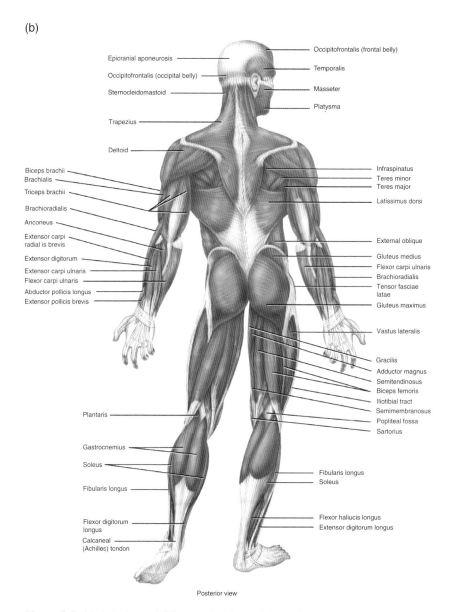

Posterior view

Figure 6.8 (a) Anterior and (b) posterior views of the major muscles of the body. Source: From Tortora and Derrickson (2017).

- Subcutaneous injections should not be administered into the intramuscular layer. Insulin injected into muscle is absorbed more rapidly, causing glucose instability and hypoglycaemia.
- Intramuscular injections should only be injected into muscle (see techniques below).
- The skin should be cleaned with an alcohol swab, such as one impregnated with 70% alcohol and chlorhexidine, prior to the injection (see Aseptic technique). IV cannula hubs should also be cleaned prior to the administration of IV medications.

Aseptic Technique

It is important to adhere to strict hand hygiene and skin cleaning prior to administering an injection. This is usually performed using a swab impregnated with isopropyl alcohol 70% and chlorhexidine 2% and leaving to dry for 30 seconds prior to injecting.

A **clean technique** is when we wash our hands and put on non-sterile gloves. We use this technique when administering injections.

We also need to be aware of the **no-touch technique**; this is where the clean hands must not contaminate our patients or any sterile equipment or patients. An example of this technique is when we have cleaned the patient's skin prior to the injection being given.

Sites on the Body for IM Injections

Gluteus Muscles

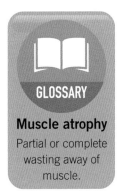

GLOSSARY

Muscle atrophy
Partial or complete wasting away of muscle.

Problems with this site include that this muscle may be atrophied in elderly, non-ambulant, and emaciated patients. This site also carries with it the danger of needle hitting the sciatic nerve and superior gluteal arteries. This site also has a low absorption rate. The maximum amount this site will hold is 4 ml in adults and 1–2 ml in children.

Deltoid Muscle

This site accommodates smaller quantities of drugs: a maximum of 0.5–1 ml.

Vastus Lateralis Muscle

This thigh muscle site is free from major nerves and blood vessels.

IM Injection Technique

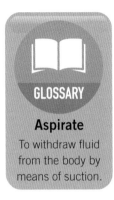

GLOSSARY

Aspirate

To withdraw fluid from the body by means of suction.

- Obtain the patient's consent.
- Aseptic procedure must be followed.
- Choose the correct site for the volume of drug.
- Prepare the skin.
- Stretch the skin and insert the needle at a 90° angle.
- Aspirate the plunger (to ascertain that you have put the needle into muscle, not a blood vessel). There is no need to aspirate if using the deltoid muscle.
- If no blood is present then inject slowly (approximately 1 ml per 10 seconds). Some drugs are given over a set time; for example, 2 ml/min.
- Wait 10 seconds, then remove the needle smoothly.
- Do not massage the site.
- Document the injection on the drug chart.

NOTE: stretching the skin first reduces the sensitivity of the nerve endings, which means less pain for the patient.

Administering 1 ml per 10 seconds seems slow, but this allows the medication to diffuse into muscle (the muscle fibres expand and absorb the solution).

Furosemide needs to be given over a set time, otherwise injection can cause speed shock and may cause tinnitus.

You must wait before removing a needle; otherwise, fluid will be drawn out along needle tract and the patient will not get the required prescription.

Z-Track Technique

Research suggests that the so-called Z-track technique results in less patient discomfort and fewer complications than the tradition IM method. Here is the Z-track technique.

- Pull the skin taut with the side of your non-dominant hand.
- The dominant hand inserts the needle.
- The dominant hand withdraws the plunger.
- After injecting, leave the needle in place for 10 seconds.
- Keep the skin taut until after the needle is removed.

This technique is used because some drugs, such as vitamin B_{12}, cause excess pain and possibly also skin discoloration.

Sites on the Body for Subcutaneous Injections

Subcutaneous injections are administered into the subcutaneous tissue rather than the muscle (Figure 6.9). Medications administered into this tissue have a slow and steady absorption and blood vessels and nerves are minimal in these areas. The sites most commonly used for subcutaneous injections are the middle outer aspect of the upper arm, the middle anterior aspect of the thigh or the anterior abdominal wall just below the umbilicus.

- Used for slow, sustained absorption of drugs.
- Up to 1–2 ml may be injected; usually with a 25 g needle for drugs such as insulin and enoxaparin sodium.
- Swab multi-use ampoules/bottles with an alcohol swab and leave to dry for 30 seconds (mode of action: dehydration).

NOTE: skin should be pinched upwards to lift the adipose tissue away from underlying muscle; otherwise the drug may be administered into muscle. Traditionally a 45° angle is used to administer into a skin fold, but for the new shorter insulin needles a 90° angle is recommended.

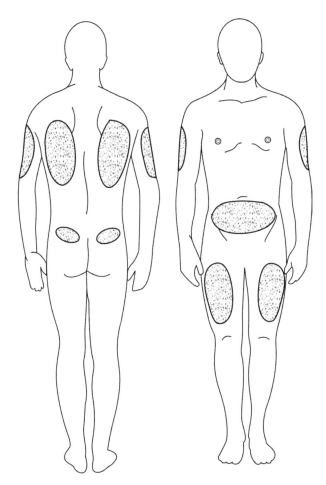

Figure 6.9 Sites recommended for subcutaneous injections (Elkin et al. 2007).

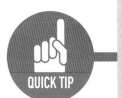
QUICK TIP

In the community, nurses may not always clean the skin for SC injections, as the alcohol swab may 'harden' the skin over time, especially for repeated insulin injections. In the hospital setting the skin is always cleaned, due to the airbourne infections and the risks of exposing the patient to a hospital-acquired infection.

SC Injection Technique

- It is not necessary to aspirate the needle after insertion: it rarely hits blood vessels.
- Inject gradually – approximately 1 ml per 10 seconds – enabling the medication to be accommodated into the site.

Preparation of a Patient
Prior to the Injection

Prior to giving an injection, a few preliminary considerations need to be made:

- Check for any allergies, and past medical history.
- Check whether the patient is needle phobic.
- Position the patient.
- Obtain consent and explain the procedure to the patient: invite questions.
- Check the patient's identity.
- Promote comfort and relaxation: *relax the muscle, as more will be pain felt if the muscle is tense.*

Disposal of Sharps

See Figure 6.10.

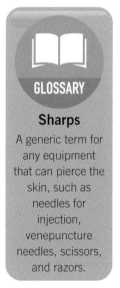

GLOSSARY

Sharps

A generic term for any equipment that can pierce the skin, such as needles for injection, venepuncture needles, scissors, and razors.

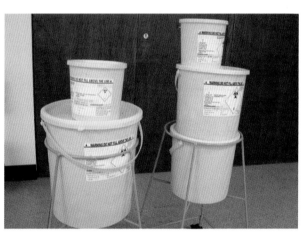

Figure 6.10 Sharps boxes.

- Take a sharps bin in a plastic tray to the patient's bedside and dispose of the needle immediately after use.
- Never re-sheath or bend needles.
- Dispose of the needle and syringe as a single unit.
- Never overfill sharps boxes.
- You will need to be aware of your area's needlestick injury helpline.
- Report all needlestick injuries.

Intradermal Injections

- Usually used for local rather than systemic drugs; for example, allergy testing, tuberculin, or local anesthetic.
- Usually performed using a 25g needle, just under the epidermis.
- Volumes used: 0.5ml or less.
- This injection site is most commonly used is the medial forearm area.
- The chosen site for diagnostic testing is the inner forearm area.
- A 10–15° angle is used, *with bevel uppermost*.
- Substance should be injected until a wheal appears on the skin surface.

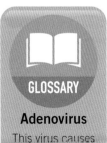

GLOSSARY

Adenovirus

This virus causes a range of illnesses such as cold-like symptoms, fever, sore-throat, bronchitis, pneumonia, diarrhoea, and conjunctivitis (pink-eye).

Vaccines

A very specific type of drug administered are vaccines for immunization. Vaccines work by stimulating your immune system to produce antibodies, exactly like it would if you had actually been exposed to the disease. After getting vaccinated, you develop immunity to that disease, all without having to get the disease first. Most vaccines are given by injection (IM) but some are given orally or nasally – sprayed directly into the nose.

Vaccines can be given for travel purposes. For example, you will need to be immunised against cholera if you wish to travel from the UK to Sub-Saharan Africa and the Middle East, South and Southeast Asia and Central America, and the Caribbean. For older individuals, they will be offered the Shingles vaccine and the influenza (flu) vaccine. There are also vaccines for childhood illnesses, such as measles. Table 6.1 shows some of the vaccines available:

Table 6.1 Vaccines.

Adenovirus	Anthrax
Cholera	Diphtheria
Hepatitis A	Hepatitis B
Japanese encephalitis	Tick-borne encephalitis
Pertussis (whooping cough)	Pneumococcal
Polio	Rabies
Rotavirus	Shingles
Smallpox	Tetanus
Human papillomavirus	Seasonal influenza
Tuberculosis	Typhoid fever
Measles	Meningococcal
Yellow fever	Varicella
Mumps	

Influenza

The flu vaccine is an example of an inactivated whole virus, as opposed to a live vaccine. This means that it is dead. It is nothing more than the protein coat of influenza with all its DNA removed. Your body will however recognise the flu virus vaccine as a foreign invader and produces antibodies against it, so that if the body encounters the virus again, it is primed to fend it off. A new version of the vaccine is developed twice a year, as the influenza virus rapidly changes, so the Scientists choose strains based on the ones they think are most likely to show up that year. You cannot get flu from the flu vaccine, but you can still get flu during the flu season, but symptoms tend to be milder as a result of the vaccination.

Coronovirus

One of the new boys on the block is the vaccine for Covid 19. These vaccines have been developed by different methods, depending on the Pharmaceutical company and Scientists. Table 6.2 shows these different types of vaccines:

Table **6.2** Covid 19 vaccine development.

Vaccine development	Information	Examples of Covid-19 vaccines
Adenoviral vaccines	These vaccines are based on weakened versions of adenoviruses, which are a group of viruses that typically infect membranes of the eyes, respiratory tract, urinary tract, intestines, and nervous system, and include the common cold. When the vaccine enters cells inside a human body, it uses the Covid genetic code to produce the spike protein. This prompts an immune response within the body, which primes the immune system to attack the coronavirus during the infection.	Oxford/Astra Zeneca Janssen (Johnson & Johnson)
mRNA Vaccines	Traditional vaccines are made up of small, inactivated doses of the whole disease-causing organism, or the proteins that it produces, which are introduced into the body to provoke the immune system into mounting a response. But mRNA vaccines trick the body into producing some of the viral proteins itself and activate T-cells to destroy the infected cells.	Pfizer/ biotech Moderna
Inactivated whole virus vaccine	Inactivated vaccines contain whole bacteria or viruses which have been killed, or small parts of the bacteria or viruses, such as proteins or sugars, which cannot cause disease.	Glaxo SmithKline (GSK)/Sanofi Pasteur Novavax
Protein adjunct Vaccine	An adjuvant (modified gene) is added to a virus to create spike proteins, which look like coronavirus but cannot replicate or cause covid-19. These nanoparticles are then injected into the body via the vaccine whereby the immune system mounts an antibody response. This has been shown to create a stronger and longer-lasting immunity against infections than the vaccine alone. The use of an adjuvant may reduce the amount of vaccine protein required per dose, which allows more vaccine doses to be produced.	Valneva

Source: Adapted from House of Commons – Science and Technology Committee. First Report of session 2019–2021

TEST YOUR KNOWLEDGE

1   Why would you inject a medication? Give four reasons.
2   How is the intramuscular route abbreviated on the prescription chart?
3   How is the subcutaneous route abbreviated on the prescription chart?
4   A drug comes in micrograms: how is this presented on the prescription chart?
5   When administering an intramuscular drug is it best practise to wear gloves? Give a reason for your answer.
6   The Covid-19 Oxford/Astra Zeneca vaccine has been developed as what type of vaccine?

KEY POINTS

- The principles of parenteral drug administration.
- Looking at syringe types and understanding the meniscus.
- Looking at the types of needle used for administering injections.
- The importance of aseptic technique.
- The sites of the body used when giving injections, and injection techniques.
- The Z-track IM injection technique.
- How to dispose of sharps.
- Looking at vaccines.

WEB RESOURCES

Government Publications

www.Publications.Parliament.UK/pa/cm5801/cmselect
www.cdc.gov/flu/prevent/keyfacts
www.nhs.uk/conditions/vaccinations/flu-influenza

REFERENCES

Elkin, M.K., Perry, A.G., and Potter, P.A. (2007). *Nursing Interventions and Clinical Skills*, 4e. St Louis, MO: Mosby.
Tortora, G.J. and Derrickson, B.H. (2017). *Tortora's Principles of Anatomy and Physiology*, 15e. John Wiley and: Sons.

Chapter 7
· · · · · · · · · · · · · · · · · · · ·
ADMINISTRATION OF RECTAL AND VAGINAL PREPARATIONS

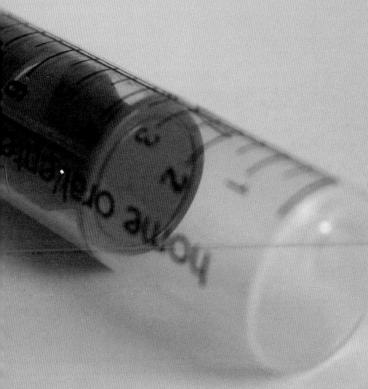

Medicine Management Skills for Nurses, Second Edition. Claire Boyd.
© 2022 John Wiley & Sons Ltd. Published 2022 by John Wiley & Sons Ltd.

LEARNING OUTCOMES

By the end of this chapter, you will have an understanding of the theory and practice of performing the clinical skill of administering rectal and vaginal preparations.

Medications administered via the rectal or vaginal routes may be a huge source of embarrassment for the patient due to the fact we are dealing with parts of the body very private to us all. It is for this reason that many patients are hesitant to report any concerns they may have with their 'nether regions', meaning their penal, vaginal, or anal areas. This may mean that they have been experiencing odour, itching, discharge, or abdominal pain due to constipation for some time. Tact, patience, and professionalism is required at all times.

I was always told, and abide by this philosophy today, that you should treat all patients as you yourself would wish to be treated and how you would wish your own loved ones to be treated.

Remember to adhere to chaperoning policies and procedures. Also, non-latex gloves should be worn when administering rectal and vaginal preparations, because if latex gloves are worn then latex will enter the body and your patient could build up a sensitivity to all latex proteins in the future.

INSERTION OF VAGINAL PESSARIES

Before the procedure begins, our patient must consent to the procedure and the medication must be prescribed on the prescription chart. We may need to ask our patient to give themselves a wash 'down below' prior to the procedure or assist them to do this (Table 7.1).

Table 7.1 Procedure for administering a vaginal pessary.

Equipment required	
Disposable gloves, swab or tissues, lubricating jelly, apron	
Intervention	**Rationale**
1 Check with patient and hospital notes for any contraindications.	To minimize risk of potential problems.
2 Explain the procedure and obtain verbal consent.	To reduce anxiety and gain consent.
3 Ensure procedure is carried out in the privacy of a cubicle or curtained area[a].	To maintain patient's privacy and dignity.
Check the following: *right medicine* is given, to the *right patient*, at the *right time*, in the *right form*, at the *right dose*.	
4 Wash hands with soap and water and put on apron and gloves.	Prevent potential contact with body fluids and minimize the risk of cross infection.
5 Position the patient in the supine position with the knees drawn up and the legs parted.	This positioning allows ease of entry into the vagina of the medication.
6 Apply lubricating jelly to a swab and wipe the pessary. Some pessaries come with an applicator, into which the pessary is inserted.	To enable the pessary to enter the vagina with minimal discomfort.
7 Insert the pessary along the posterior vaginal wall and into the top of the vagina.	To ensure the patient's comfort and for medication to reach correct site.
8 Wipe away any excess lubricating jelly from the patient's vulva with a swab or tissue.	To minimise patient discomfort.
9 Make the patient comfortable.	To minimize patient discomfort.
10 Remove gloves and apron (into clinical waste bag) and you're your hands.	To minimize risk of cross infection.
11 Record the administration of the medication on the prescription chart.	To keep accurate documentation.

[a]Where available and appropriate insertion of pessaries should be performed in a side room to protect the privacy and dignity of the patient.

INSERTION OF RECTAL MEDICINES

Drugs can be administered via the rectum:

- In a solid form as a suppository; these drugs melt at body temperature,
- As a solution, suspension or foam; these drugs are known as enemas.

The absorption rate of the rectum can be rapid, but in the presence of faeces this can be slowed. On the continent, many drugs are administered via the rectal route.

As with all healthcare issues, patients should be taught self care and to self-administrate their suppositories, but this may not always be feasible.

Patients' stools are assessed using the Bristol Stool Chart, which is shown in Figure 7.1.

Laxatives are administered to evacuate the rectum and should be retained for at least 20 minutes to be effective.

Prior to administration of medication via the rectal route, a digital rectal examination should be performed.

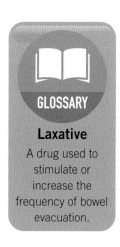

GLOSSARY

Laxative
A drug used to stimulate or increase the frequency of bowel evacuation.

Digital Rectal Examination

A digital rectal examination (or DRE) may be used as part of a nursing assessment to establish the presence of stool in the rectum; a care plan will outline the intervention required for the patient. A DRE is performed:

- To assess presence of stool in the rectum, amount and consistency,
- To assess the need for rectal medication,
- To evaluate the efficacy of interventions/medication,
- To assess anal tone and contraction and to what degree.

Constipation

Constipation can affect any age and gender, but it is more common in the older population. Any of us may develop constipation when we are unwell or admitted to hospital as we may not be able to move around as well, sweat more, drink less fluid and eat differently (perhaps with less fibre)

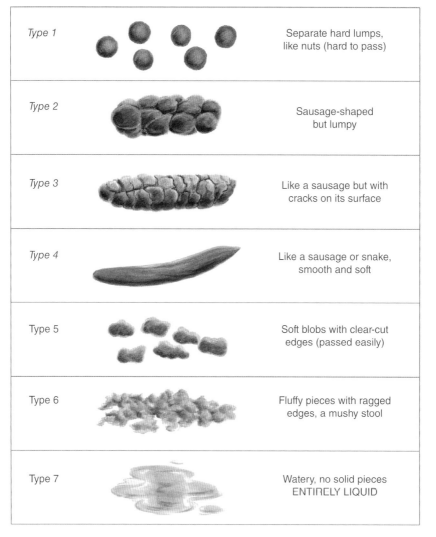

Type 1		Separate hard lumps, like nuts (hard to pass)
Type 2		Sausage-shaped but lumpy
Type 3		Like a sausage but with cracks on its surface
Type 4		Like a sausage or snake, smooth and soft
Type 5		Soft blobs with clear-cut edges (passed easily)
Type 6		Fluffy pieces with ragged edges, a mushy stool
Type 7		Watery, no solid pieces ENTIRELY LIQUID

Figure 7.1 Bristol stool chart. Source: Permission to reproduce this image is granted by North Bristol NHS Trust and University Hospitals Bristol NHS Foundation Trust.

than we would at home. There are also medicines that are associated with constipation, such as:

- Anticholinergics, such as oxybutynin
- Antiepileptics, such as Carbamazepine

- Antidepressants, such as Amitriptyline
- Antiparkinsonians, such as Procyclidine
- Antipsychotics, such as Haloperidol
- Calcium Supplements, such as Calcium gluconate
- Diuretics, such as Bendrofluazide
- Iron tablets, such as Ferrous Sulphate
- Opiates, such as Codeine Phosphate
- Aluminium Antacids, such as Aluminium hydroxide.

Constipation may make it hard to pass a bowel movement and may look like numbers 1–3 on the Bristol Stool Chart (Figure 7.1). This should not be treated lightly as it leads to feelings of being bloated, lethargic, and very unwell. The patient may be prescribed an enema or suppositories to relieve their symptoms.

Administration of Enemas and Suppositories

A DRE should be carried out to assess for faecal loading and for abnormalities including blood, pain, and obstruction. Indications for insertion of suppositories or enemas include:

- evacuation of faecal matter from the bowel,
- treatment of inflammatory bowel conditions,
- neurogenic bowel dysfunction as part of a regular-bowel management programme,
- spinal cord injuries as part of a regular-bowel management programme,
- drug administration as an alternative to the oral route, to be absorbed for systemic effect.

Autonomic Dysreflexia

Extra care must be taken with performing rectal procedures on spinally injured patients, as a condition called autonomic dysreflexia (or ADR) may be initiated. This condition is also known as hyperreflexia. Some clinical areas only permit experienced staff to undertake these clinical procedures on spinally injured patients.

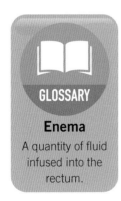

GLOSSARY

Enema
A quantity of fluid infused into the rectum.

DID YOU KNOW?

A small number of patients who have had a severe stroke, or who have Parkinson's disease, multiple sclerosis, cerebral palsy, or spinal bifida may also be susceptible to ADR.

Care and Management of Autonomic Dysreflexia

ADR is a syndrome unique to patients with spinal cord injury at the level of the sixth thoracic vertebrae or above. It may also affect people with neurological disease or injury, such as Guillain- Barre Syndrome, Multiple Sclerosis etc. It is a sudden, potentially lethal rise in blood pressure and is often triggered by acute pain or harmful stimulus below the level of the injury.

It should always be treated as a medical emergency; if left untreated, it can be fatal due to the risk of cerebral haemorrhage, seizure, or cardiac arrest. The condition arises as a result of an autonomic (sympathetic) reflex as a response to pain or discomfort (noxious stimuli) perceived below the level of the lesion.

The reflex creates a massive vasoconstriction below the level of the lesion causing a pathological rise in blood pressure that can be life-threatening if allowed to continue unchecked.

Patients who have been discharged from a spinal injury unit should never have their bowel management programme altered without first consulting with the spinal injury unit that other methods of evacuation are suitable (National Policies Safety Agency).

The risk assessment is part of a bowel-dysfunction assessment and a full medical history should be considered prior to any bowel-related procedures.

Manifestations of ADR include:

- Severe hypertension,
- Bradycardia,

- 'Pounding' headache,
- Flushed or 'blotchy' skin above the level of lesion,
- Pallor below the level of lesion,
- Profuse sweating above the level of lesion,
- Shortness of breath.

Common causes:

- Any painful or noxious stimuli below the level of the injury,
- Distended bladder (usually due to catheter blockage or another form of Bladder outlet obstruction),
- Distended bowel (usually due to a full rectum, constipation or impaction),
- Skin problems/in-growing toenail,
- Fracture below the level of the lesion,
- Labour/childbirth,
- Ejaculation.

Actions to take:

- Sit the patient up (where possiblc) to induce an element of postural hypotension.
- Ensure there is adequate urinary drainage (change the catheter if necessary, do not give a bladder washout/ instillation).
- Empty the rectum by digital removal of faeces (local anaesthetic gel should be used).
- Blood pressure should be treated until the cause is found and eliminated (administer a proprietary vasodilator, e.g. nifedipine, as prescribed).
- If unable to locate cause, or symptoms persist, get help immediately.

ADR can usually be remedied easily by the removal of the cause of the painful stimuli, use of local anaesthetic and/or use of a vasodilator.

Procedural Steps for DRE

There are circumstances to consider where extra care is required and exclusions and contra-indications. Before undertaking DRE, abnormalities of the perineal and perianal areas should be observed, looking for: rectal prolapse, haemorrhoids, anal skin tags, wounds, dressings, discharge, anal lesions, gaping anus, skin condition, bleeding, faecal matter, infestation and foreign bodies (Table 7.2).

Table 7.2 Procedure for DRE.

Equipment required
Disposable latex free gloves, incontinence sheet/pad, wipes, lubricant (e.g. KY jelly), clinical waste bag, plastic apron.

Intervention	Rationale
1 Check with patient and hospital notes for any contraindications.	To minimize risk of potential problems.
2 Explain the procedure and obtain verbal consent.	To reduce anxiety and gain consent.
3 Ensure procedure is carried out in the privacy of a cubicle or curtained area[a].	To maintain patient's privacy and dignity.
4 Wash your hands with soap and water and put on apron and double gloves.	Prevent potential contact with body fluids and minimize the risk of cross infection.
5 Position the patient on their left side with their back next to the edge of the bed, and their knees flexed. Place an absorbent pad under the patient and cover the patient with a sheet.	This positioning allows ease of entry into the rectum following the natural curve of the colon.
6 Examine the perianal area for any abnormalities before proceeding.	To ensure that it is safe to proceed.
7 Reassure the patient throughout the procedure.	To avoid unnecessary stress or embarrassment and ensure continued consent.
8 Lubricate gloved index finger and insert gently into the rectum. NOTE: your nails must be kept short.	To minimise patient discomfort and avoid anal mucosal trauma.
9 Assess for the presence of faecal matter using the Bristol Stool Scale.	To check for the presence of faecal matter and to establish the consistency of the stool.

(*Continued*)

Table **7.2** (*Continued*)

Intervention	Rationale
10 Slowly withdraw your finger from patient's rectum when finished. Check for presence of faeces or blood on the glove.	To minimize patient discomfort.
11 Remove top glove and dispose of it in a clinical waste bag.	To minimize risk of cross infection.
12 Wipe residual lubricating gel from anal area.	To ensure the patient's comfort and avoid anal excoriation.
13 Dispose of gloves, apron and equipment into a clinical waste bag and wash hands.	To prevent cross infection.
14 Ensure that the patient is comfortable and observe for any adverse reactions.	To and minimise embarrassment and note adverse reactions.
15 Record findings in nursing documentation and communicate findings with medical team if appropriate. Consistency, volume, date, and time should all be recorded appropriately.	To ensure correct care and continuity of care.

*Where available and appropriate DRE and insertion of suppositories and enemas should be performed in a side room to protect the privacy and dignity of the patient, and protect other patients from potential malodour.

Procedural Steps for Administration of Enemas and Suppositories

There are circumstances to consider where extra care is required and exclusions and contra-indications. Before inserting enemas or suppositories, abnormalities of the perineal and perianal area should be observed as per DRE. Special precautions also need to be assessed: recent colorectal surgery, malignancy (or other pathology) of the perianal region and low platelet count (Table 7.3).

Table 7.3 Procedure for administering enemas and suppositories.

Equipment required	
Disposable latex free gloves, incontinence sheet/pad, wipes, lubricant (e.g. KY jelly), clinical waste bag, plastic apron, suppository or enema as prescribed by medic or nurse prescriber.	

Intervention	Rationale
1 Obtain verbal consent and document it.	To reduce anxiety and gain consent.
2 Collect and prepare the necessary equipment.	To ensure procedure is conducted in an efficient and timely manner, thus reducing anxiety.
3 Take the patient's pulse rate at rest prior to and during the procedure.	To record baseline pulse and monitor for changes.
4 Take blood pressure in spinally injured patients prior to, during and at the end of the procedure.	To record baseline pulse and monitor for changes.
5 Prepare the patient; assist with removing clothing from waist down, help in positioning patient in a left lateral position, knees flexed, taking into consideration the normal line of the sigmoid colon.	This positioning allows ease of entry into the rectum following the natural curve of the colon.
6 Protect bedding and mattress and wash hands with soap and water.	To maintain infection control procedures and patient dignity.
7 Observe the anal area and put on gloves and apron.	To ensure that it is safe to proceed. To prevent potential contact with body fluids and minimize the risk of cross infection.
8 Lubricate the gloved index finger; inform the patient that you are about to perform the procedure.	To minimise patient discomfort and avoid anal mucosal trauma.
9 Gain patient co-operation by asking the patient to relax prior to insertion of index or middle finger.	To avoid unnecessary stress or embarrassment and ensure continued consent.
10 Insert the gloved finger into the anus slowly and on into the rectum.	To minimise patient discomfort and avoid anal mucosal trauma.

(*Continued*)

Table 7.3 (*Continued*)

Intervention	Rationale
11 Assess for faecal matter and document the amount and consistency using the Bristol Stool Scale. Assess the need for medication.	To establish rectal loading and the consistency of the stool.
12 Lubricate the blunt end of the suppository or the tube tip of the enema (after cap has been removed); inform the patient that you are about to perform the procedure, then insert the suppository/enema via the anus into the rectum.	Inserting the suppository blunt end first allows the anal sphincter to assist with insertion.
13 Clean anal area; remove gel by wiping residual from area to ensure that it does not cause irritation or soreness.	To maintain cleanliness. To leave patient comfortable.
14 Dispose of equipment as per local policy into a clinical waste bag.	To prevent cross infection.
15 Help patient to get up and dressed and into a comfortable position, offer toileting facilities as appropriate.	To maintain dignity and to minimise embarrassment.
16 Document the procedure fully on completion.	To establish effectiveness of procedure. To ensure continuity of care.

TEST YOUR KNOWLEDGE

1   A female patient has vulval candidiasis. The drug prescribed for this condition, clotrimazole, comes in the format of 100 mg pessaries. The medic writes this up as 'Clotrimazole. Insert 400 mg for 3 nights'. Describe the procedure for insertion to a student nurse.

2   What is ADR? What is the treatment for this condition?

KEY POINTS

- The procedure for administering vaginal pessaries and rectal medications.
- The procedure for conducting a DRE.
- Understanding medications associated with constipation.
- The care and management of ADR.

WEB RESOURCES

BNF Adults: www.bnf.nice.org.uk
BNF Children: www.bnfc.nice.org.uk
The Royal Marsden Clinical Nursing Procedures:
www.rmmonline.co.uk/manual
You will need to register and log in.
National Patient Safety Agency: www.npsa.org.uk
Spinal Injuries Association www.spinal.co.uk

Chapter 8
· ·
ADMINISTRATION OF TOPICAL PREPARATIONS

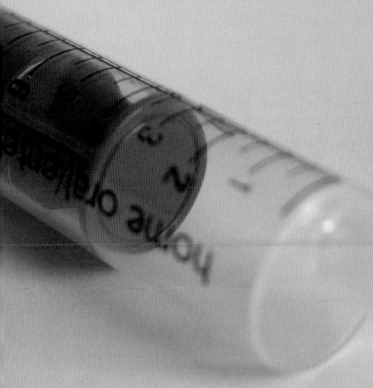

Medicine Management Skills for Nurses, Second Edition. Claire Boyd.
© 2022 John Wiley & Sons Ltd. Published 2022 by John Wiley & Sons Ltd.

LEARNING OUTCOMES

By the end of this chapter you will have an understanding of the theory and practice of performing the clinical skill of administering topical preparations.

The topical route of drug administration has become a popular means of drug application due to the fact that it can be made available almost directly to the intended site of action and the risk of systemic side effects may be reduced. Topical drug administration includes medications such as:

- Eye drops for the treatment of glaucoma,
- Application of topical steroids in the management of dermatitis,
- Bronchodilators in the treatment of asthma,
- Pessaries containing clotrimazole in the treatment of vaginal candidiasis (see Chapter 7).

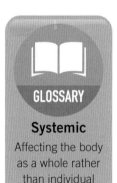

GLOSSARY

Systemic

Affecting the body as a whole rather than individual parts and organs.

Some topical medications have a local effect – for example, hydrocortisone creams and ointments prescribed for eczema and dermatitis – treating the affected area only. Some medications go through the skin into the bloodstream to work around the body; for example, anti-inflammatory gels. This is known as a systemic effect.

The topical route also applies to patches, such as hormone-replacement therapy (or HRT) and nicotine patches. These are known as transdermal patches. They have a systemic rather than a local effect in the body (these are dealt with below).

Due to the fact that medication applied in cream, gel, or patch format travels through the skin and enters the bloodstream, if an anti-inflammatory cream is applied to the skin then an oral anti-inflammatory drug cannot also be administered, as there will be a risk of overdose. Some topical medications have a more localised effect.

As with all medication administration, it must be recorded that a topical medication has been administered.

Storage is also an important factor, as some medications may need to be stored in the fridge, or away from direct sunlight. Some of these medications may be presented in brown or blue bottles, so that the light does not damage the active ingredients inside.

APPLYING CREAMS AND OINTMENTS

Some creams are used as part of a skin integrity programme, such as pressure-relief care, and you will be advised to use just a small amount. Other prescribed medications, such as anti-inflammatories and steroidal creams, may need to be applied in a much more accurate dose.

Many pharmaceutical products for topical application express the active ingredients as a percentage weight for weight; for example, 1% w/w hydrocortisone cream.

Some areas in the community tend to apply these creams according to 'fingertip' unit measurements. Of course, this does depend on the nozzle size of the tube and the general practitioner (GP)'s and/or pharmacy instructions.

Fingertip Units

One fingertip unit is the distance from the tip of an adult index finger to the first crease of that finger (Figure 8.1).

Tables 8.1 and 8.2 give you a rough guide of how much cream or ointment to use for an adult and a child.

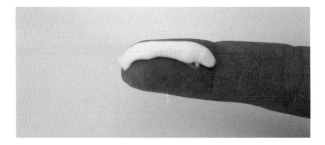

Figure 8.1 One fingertip unit.

Table 8.1 Amount of cream to use for an adult.

Affected body area	Quantity of cream or ointment
Both sides of one hand	One fingertip unit
One foot	Two fingertip units
One arm	Three fingertip units
One leg	Six fingertip units
Chest and abdomen	Seven fingertip units
Back and buttocks	Seven fingertip units
Face and neck	Two and a half fingertip units

Table 8.2 Amount of cream to use for a child.

Area	3–6 mo	1–2 yr	3–5 yr	6–10 yr
Face and neck	One fingertip unit	One and a half fingertip units	One and a half fingertip units	Two fingertip units
Arm and hand	One fingertip unit	One and a half fingertip units	Two fingertip units	Two and a half fingertip units
Leg and foot	One and a half fingertip units	Two fingertip units	Three fingertip units	Four and a half fingertip units
Trunk (front)	One fingertip unit	Two fingertip units	Three fingertip units	Three and a half fingertip units
Trunk (back)	One and a half fingertip units	Three fingertip units	Three and a half fingertip units	Five fingertip units

Skin Condition

Applying creams and ointments to the skin gives us the ideal opportunity to assess our patient. Many systemic diseases manifest their diagnostic features in the skin, and act as a barometer for an individual's general health (Table 8.3).

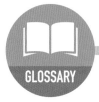
GLOSSARY

Oedema/oedematous
Excessive accumulation of fluid in the bodily tissues.

Table 8.3 Systemic diseases manifesting their diagnostic features in the skin.

Systemic disease	Skin manifestation
Congested cardiac failure	Cyanosed, oedematous
Hypertension	May be highly coloured
Chronic obstructive airways disease	Dusky hue or bright pink
Hypoglycaemia	Profusely sweating
Chronic renal failure	Yellow-brown
Iron deficiency anaemia	Pale
Pernicious anaemia	Pale lemon-tinted
Viral diseases	Rashes, itching

Applying Creams and Ointments (Table 8.4)

Table 8.4 Procedure for applying creams and ointments.

Equipment required	
Disposable gloves, apron, medication	
Intervention	**Rationale**
1 Check with patient and hospital notes for any contraindications.	To minimise risk of potential problems
2 Explain the procedure and obtain verbal consent.	To reduce anxiety and gain consent
3 Remove clothing where medication is to be applied and clean skin if necessary. Any previous cream should be completely removed. Creams should not be used immediately before or after bathing. This may require careful planning.	To allow medication to reach area that is being treated, on clean, dry skin
Check the following: *right medicine* is given, to the *right patient,* at the *right time,* in the *right form,* at the *right dose.*	

(*Continued*)

Table 8.4 (*Continued*)

Intervention	Rationale
4 Wash hands with soap and water and put on apron and gloves.	To minimise the risk of cross infection and to enable the medication not to be absorbed through your own skin
5 Position the patient, either sitting or lying down.	For patient comfort during procedure
6 Apply the cream gently following the line of the hairs: rubbing downwards (but with certain medical conditions, such as oedema, one needs to rub upwards to help the lymph drainage).	To avoid folliculitis
7 Remove gloves and apron (place in clinical waste bag) and wash hands.	To minimise risk of cross infection
8 Make the patient comfortable.	To minimise patient discomfort
9 Record the administration of the medication on the prescription chart.	To keep accurate documentation

Most jars of creams may only keep for one month after opening and tubes for three months: you will need to read the pharmacist's instructions. It is good practice therefore to write on the jar or tube the date that it was opened, as packaging may have a manufacturers date many years in advance just stating how long the contents will remain stable without opening. This is the best-before date.

Jars and tubs should not be used for more than one patient, as this will be an infection risk.

TRANSDERMAL PATCHES

The transdermal patch was developed in the early 1980s and has since become a popular means of introducing drugs into the systemic circulation through the skin. Some of the drugs you may see administered by this means include:

- hyoscine-based products for the treatment of nausea,
- glyceryl trinitrate for the prophylactic treatment of angina,

- fentanyl for the treatment of chronic pain,
- oestrogens for hormone-replacement treatments.

NOTE: some individuals may experience local skin reactions.

Applying a Transdermal Patch

Before applying a transdermal patch the following points need to be addressed.

- Ensure the skin is dry and clean.
- The patch should be applied to a hairless patch of skin.
- When changing the patch, always apply to a different site to avoid sore skin and rashes.
- Observe skin condition.
- Always wash your hands before and after the procedure.
- Wear gloves when applying the patch.
- Dispose of the old patch by folding in half.
- Document on the prescription chart in the usual way.

EYE DROPS

Eye drops should always be applied to clean eyes (Figure 8.2), so they may need to be cleaned with saline or water prior to the procedure, wiping from the inside corner outwards. Gloves should be worn for the administration of eye drops, especially if the patient has an eye infection.

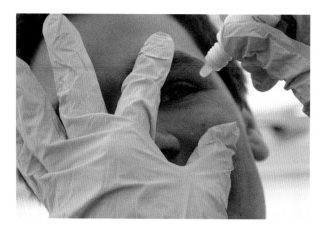

Figure 8.2 Applying eye drops.

Sometimes only one eye will need to be treated, so read the prescription carefully. Other considerations need to be adhered to, such as checking to see whether your patient is wearing contact lens (which will need to be removed) or if the patient has a glass eye.

Eye drops may come with a glass dropper or in a container whereby you just need to squeeze the drops into the eye. Try not to contaminate the container by touching the eye; if this does occur, wipe the container. Always put the cap back on as soon as the drops have been administered to prevent the solution from becoming contaminated. It is also best practise to write the date the bottle was opened, with the same rationale as for creams and lotions, as once opened the contents may only remain stable for 28 days. It is also usual practise to have two bottles in a hospital setting, one for the left eye and one for the right eye. This information should also be written on the bottle or ampoule.

Eye Conditions

Some of the common eye conditions:

- Conjunctivitis: bacterial or viral,
- Corneal ulceration,
- Glaucoma,
- Foreign body in the eye.

Inflammatory eyelid disorders:

- Blepharitis (lid may become inflamed and crusty),
- Orbital cellulitis (often results from a spread of infection from the sinuses),
- Allergy (may occur as a result of direct contact from cosmetics),
- Viral infections (may occur due to infections such as herpes simplex or herpes zoster viruses),
- Drooping of the eyelid, or ptosis (may indicate the presence of myasthenia gravis).

Lacrimal disorders:

- Excessive tear production (often watering of the eye due to blockage of the lacrimal sac or nasolacrimal duct),

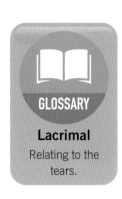

GLOSSARY

Lacrimal
Relating to the tears.

- Dry eye syndrome (deficiency of either the aqueous or mucin component of the tear film causing discomfort).

Glaucoma

This condition is characterised by a raised intra-ocular pressure which leads to a cupping and degeneration of the optic disc. It may be treated with:

- betaxolol hydrochloride drops,
- timolol maleate drops,
- antibacterial eye drops:
  - chloramphenicol 0.5% drops,
  - chloramphenicol eye ointment 1%,
  - gentamicin drops 0.3%.

Applying Eye Drops (Table 8.5)

Table 8.5 Procedure for applying eye drops.

Equipment required	
Disposable gloves, apron, medication, cotton wool, tissues, sterile water, or normal saline to clean	
Intervention	**Rationale**
1 Check with patient and hospital notes for any contraindications.	To minimise risk of potential problems
2 Explain the procedure and obtain verbal consent.	To reduce anxiety and gain consent
3 Check the expiry date of the eye drops. Write on bottle the date that it was opened, and write L or R for left or right eye. In the community generally only one bottle of medication is prescribed if both eyes require treatment.	To prevent cross-contamination
Check the following: *right medicine* is given, to the *right patient,* at the *right time,* in the *right form,* at the *right dose.*	

(*Continued*)

Table 8.5 (*Continued*)

Intervention	Rationale
4 Wash hands with soap and water and put on apron and gloves.	To minimise the risk of cross infection and to enable the medication not to be absorbed through your own skin
5 Position patient either sitting or lying down, with the head tilted backwards. Gently warm the bottle in your hands if it is stored in fridge. *Shake contents.* Wipe the patient's eye from the nasal corner outwards with sterile water or normal saline before applying the drops.	For patient comfort during procedure to prevent cross-contamination
6 Gently pull the patient's eyelid down. Hold the dropper above the eye and squeeze one drop inside the lower lid. Avoid touching the dropper tip against the eyelid or contaminating it. Do not drop medication from a height into the eyeball, as this can be extremely painful.	For patient comfort during procedure to prevent cross-contamination
7 Release the eyelid and encourage the patient to blink a few times to ensure the eye is covered with the liquid. Wipe away any excess with a clean tissue. Wait a few moments before adding additional drops to allow the drops to be absorbed. *Discard the medication after 1 month,* as it becomes a source of infection. If the tip touches eye then you need to wash the tip.	For patient comfort to prevent cross-contamination
8 Remove gloves and apron (place in a clinical waste bag) and wash hands.	To minimise risk of cross infection
9 Make the patient comfortable.	To minimise patient discomfort
10 Record the administration of the medication on the prescription chart.	To keep accurate documentation

EYE OINTMENT

If eye ointment and eye drops are to be administered, it is usual for the eye ointment to be applied after the eye drops, as when wiping away any excess liquid after applying drops you may inadvertently wipe away the ointment as well. Eye ointments are usually discarded after one month of opening (28 days). On a hot day, once the cap is removed, the contents may spill out. It may be possible to place the tube in a glass of cold water to minimise this effect, but speak to the pharmacist first. Some tubes require piercing to open: the cap usually contains a piercer for this purpose, set deep within the cap to prevent any needlestick-type injuries.

Applying Eye Ointment

This is the same procedure as applying eye drops, but the following considerations need to be addressed.

- The tube may need to be pierced prior to use.
- Squeeze about 2 cm of the ointment along the inside of the lower eyelid.
- Ask the patient to close their eyes and blink several times to allow the ointment to spread over the surface of the eye.
- Wipe away any excess.
- When they open their eye, their vision may be blurred. Reassure them that blinking will clear this.

EAR DROPS

As with all the drops, when administering we need to think about our patient/service user. We need to get them into the best position for the administration of the medication. Therefore, before we begin the procedure, we need to assist the patient, or ask them to tilt their head back or to one side. As they may be in this position for a little while, it may be better to get them to actually lie down so that they are comfortable. Some patients may ask for a small piece of cotton wool to go into the ear after the procedure. We may need to explain to them that this is an infection risk, as the cotton wool may be forgotten about. Also, the cotton wool will absorb the medication, instead of treating the ear. When we apply ear drops, we want the medication to go down the ear canal as far as possible, rather than to sit in the external ear. Again, the contents are usually discarded one month after opening (28 days).

Ear Conditions

Some common ear conditions include:

- Otitis externa, which may be treated with chloramphenicol drops,
- Acute otitis media, which may be treated with systemic antibacterial drugs,
- Chronic otitis media, which may require systemic treatment with amoxicillin and/or surgery.

Applying Ear Drops (Table 8.6)

Table 8.6 Procedure for applying ear drops.

Equipment required	
Disposable gloves, apron, medication	
Intervention	**Rationale**
1 Check with patient and hospital notes for any contraindications.	To minimise risk of potential problems
2 Explain the procedure and obtain verbal consent.	To reduce anxiety and gain consent
3 Check the expiry date of the ear drops. Write the date opened on the bottle, and L or R for left or right ear. In the community generally only one bottle of medication is prescribed if both ears require treatment.	To prevent cross-contamination
Check the following: *right medicine* is given, to the *right patient*, at the *right time*, in the *right form*, at the *right dose*.	

Intervention	Rationale
4 Wash hands with soap and water and put on apron and gloves.	To minimise the risk of cross infection and to enable the medication not to be absorbed through your own skin
5 Position patient either sitting or lying down, with the head tilted backwards and to one side. Gently warm the bottle in your hands if it is stored in the fridge. *Shake contents.*	For patient comfort during procedure To prevent cross-contamination
6 Administer the drops, and replace the top immediately. Leave the head tilted for approximately 5 min and the wipe away the excess.	For patient comfort during procedure To prevent cross-contamination To allow medication to reach area being treated
7 *Discard the medication after one month* as it could become a source of infection. If the tip touches ear you need to wash the tip. Use ear drops for the full length of treatment. Avoid getting water in the ear while the patient/service user is having ear drops.	For patient comfort To prevent cross-contamination
8 Remove gloves and apron (place in a clinical waste bag) and wash hands.	To minimise risk of cross infection
9 Make the patient comfortable.	To minimise patient discomfort
10 Record the administration of the medication on the prescription chart.	To keep accurate documentation

NOSE DROPS

Nasal drops often come with long tubes so that the medication can be applied to the very back of the nasal cavity. Some are provided as pressurised sprays. Whichever device is used it should be cleaned after each use. Once opened, these medications very often only have a short shelf life, so you will need to check the manufacturer's instructions.

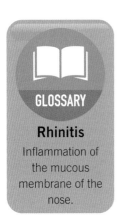

Nose Conditions

Common nose conditions include:

- Nasal allergy, allergic rhinitis: may be treated with beclomethasone dipropionate drops,
- Nasal congestion, common cold: may be treated with xylometazoline hydrochloride,
- Nasal infection: may be treated with chlorhexidine hydrochloride 0.1%, neomycin sulphate 0.5% (such as Naseptin).

Applying Nose Drops or Sprays (Table 8.7)

Table 8.7 Procedure for applying nose drops or sprays.

Equipment required	
Disposable gloves, apron, medication, tissues	
Intervention	**Rationale**
1 Check with patient and hospital notes for any contraindications.	To minimise risk of potential problems
2 Explain the procedure and obtain verbal consent.	To reduce anxiety and gain consent
3 Check the expiry date of the medication. Write the date opened on the bottle.	To prevent cross-contamination
Check the following: *right medicine* is given, to the *right patient,* at the *right time,* in the *right form,* at the *right dose.*	
4 Wash hands with soap and water and put on apron and gloves.	To minimise the risk of cross infection and to enable the medication not to be absorbed through your own skin
5 Position the patient either sitting or lying down, with the head tilted backwards, nares facing upwards. *Shake contents.*	For patient comfort during procedure To prevent cross-contamination

Intervention	Rationale
6 Administer the drops/spray by squeezing one drop at a time inside the nare/s. Ask the patient to sniff, thus drawing liquid up into the nasal cavity. Ask the patient to move the head to right and left (if able). Replace the top immediately and wipe away the excess.	To allow medication to reach area being treated To prevent cross-contamination
7 If the tip touches the nose you will need to wash the tip. Encourage the patient to rest for a short while to ensure that the medication does not drip out immediately.	To prevent cross-contamination
8 Remove gloves and apron (place in a clinical waste bag) and wash hands.	To minimise risk of cross infection
9 Make the patient comfortable.	To minimise patient discomfort
10 Record the administration of the medication on the prescription chart.	To keep accurate documentation

TEST YOUR KNOWLEDGE

1 You have been asked to use the fingertip unit measurement scale. How is this measured?

2 How much cream needs to be applied to one side of the hand, using the fingertip measurement scale?

3 If a tube of steroidal cream states that the expiry date is 2032 and was opened six months ago, can we still use it on our patient?

4 What is the procedure to administer eye drops?

KEY POINTS

- How to apply topical creams and ointments using the fingertip unit.
- The principles of applying transdermal patches.
- Looking at common eye conditions and the principles of applying eye drops and ointments.
- Looking at some common ear conditions and the principles of applying ear drops.
- Looking at some common conditions affecting the nose and the principles of applying nose drops and sprays.

WEB RESOURCES

BNF Adults: www.bnf.nice.org.uk
BNF Children: www.bnfc.nice.org.uk
The Royal Marsden Clinical Nursing Procedures:
   www.rmmonline.co.uk/manual
You will need to register and log in.

Chapter 9
. . . .
ADMINISTRATION OF INHALATION MEDICATIONS AND NEBULISERS

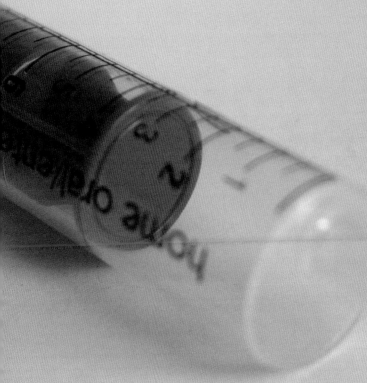

Medicine Management Skills for Nurses, Second Edition. Claire Boyd.
© 2022 John Wiley & Sons Ltd. Published 2022 by John Wiley & Sons Ltd.

LEARNING OUTCOMES

By the end of this chapter you will have an understanding of the theory and practice of performing the clinical skill of administering inhalation medications and nebulisers.

Inhalation allows the delivery of a range of drugs, with the aim of a localised therapeutic effect. This may be achieved by:

- Nebulisation,
- Aerosolisation.

The medication is delivered in a very fine format.

Some of the medical conditions for which we may administer drugs via this route are:

- Asthma,
- Chronic obstructive pulmonary disease (also known as COPD; examples include bronchitis and emphysema),
- Cystic fibrosis,
- HIV/AIDS,
- Symptom relief in palliative care.

NEBULISATION

This involves passage of air or oxygen driven through a solution of a drug, via a compressor machine, which may be electric or battery-operated. The resulting mist is inhaled via a face mask or mouthpiece. Nebulisers are used to deliver higher doses of a drug to the airways than a standard inhaler. Bronchodilators and antibiotics, among others, may be delivered in this way. Things to remember include:

- Masks and mouthpieces should be washed in warm, soapy water after use and dried well. They should be changed every three months,

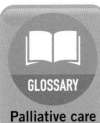

GLOSSARY

Palliative care

Care given to improve the quality of life for patients who have a serious or life-threatening disease.

- Before the next administration air should be blown through the equipment for 10 seconds to remove any residual fluids,
- Machined should be serviced regularly.

Medications are administered over 5–10 minutes from the nebuliser device. In the hospital environment nebulised drugs are administered via the piped oxygen system or via large oxygen or air cylinders.

AEROSOLISATION

Inhalers are medical devices that allow medicine to be administered directly to the lungs. They come in a variety of different shapes and forms. Some of the medications administered via inhalation include:

- Steroids,
- Insulin,
- Antibiotics,
- Bronchodilators, which are used to alleviate the symptoms of asthma, chronic bronchitis and emphysema, by opening air passages in the lungs to allow easier breathing.

While they are not a cure for asthma, bronchodilators can temporarily relieve the classic symptoms of the disease: wheezing, coughing, shortness of breath and tightness of the chest. They can also prevent bronchospasm when taken shortly before exercise.

Exubera: Inhalable Insulin

This is an alternative to daily insulin injection for patients with Type 2 diabetes. It is a powdered form of recombinant human insulin that is inhaled. It will not replace injections needed in Type 1 diabetes and is relatively new to the market.

Asthma and COPD

Asthma is a chronic inflammatory condition of the airways that affects 5.2 million individuals in the UK. Poor inhaler technique has been estimated to cost the UK National Health Service (NHS) £61 million a year, due to hospital admissions that may have been avoided. It is essential that patients are engaged with their asthma treatment for better compliance to be reached.

There are two main types of inhaler used in asthma and COPD: relievers and preventers.

Reliever Inhalers

These devices may be blue or green and the medicine opens up the airway passages to make breathing easier. An example of an aerosol inhalation reliever is salbutamol (or albuterol). Adults are usually prescribed one or two puffs four times a day. Each puff equates to 100 μg (therefore two puffs = 200 μg). Children are usually prescribed one puff, increased to two puffs if necessary, up to four times per day.

Preventer Inhalers

Preventers are used every day to reduce the inflammation in the lungs and slow down damage to the lungs over the long term. They should be used regularly, even if the individual user feels well. They usually contain steroids, for example beclomethasone, budesonide and fluticasone. Steroid inhalers are usually coloured brown or maroon. After use of a steroidal inhaler, the mouth should be rinsed with water to avoid a sore mouth or hoarse voice.

Combined Treatment with Reliever and Preventer

If a reliever and preventer are used, we need to inform our patient/service user it is best to use the reliever first. This is because the reliever opens up the airways first so that the preventer medicine can get down to the bottom of the lungs. Some inhalers, such as Seretide, contain a reliever and a preventer and should be used regularly.

Inhaler Devices

What different types of inhaler devices will our patients and service users be using?

- Metered-dose inhaler: these have a gas propellant so do not need much suck, but still need co-ordination.
- Breath-actuated aerosol inhaler: triggered by the act of breathing in.
- Powder forms of medication: these are sucked into the lungs on breathing in, avoiding the need for an aerosol gas.
- Spacer device: these allow the medication to 'hang' in the spacer until the patient breathes it in.

Some branded inhalers are discussed in more detail below.

Spacer Devices

Individuals can be taught to use aerosol inhalers effectively, but some, such as older people and small children, may find it difficult to use them, as co-ordinating the squeezing of the device and inhaling the measured burst of the medication can be difficult. In such cases a spacer device (Figure 9.1) may be necessary. A spacer is a large two-part container made of plastic that has a mouthpiece at one end and a hole at the other. The mouthpiece is the part used to inhale the respiratory medication. The hole at the other end is where the inhaler attaches. Spacer devices come in a variety of sizes, the larger devices with a one-way valve often being the most effective.

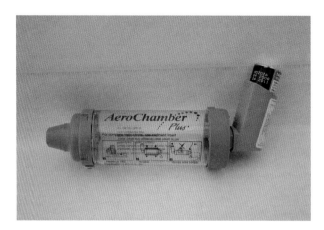

Figure 9.1 A spacer device.

Spacer devices remove the need for co-ordination between the valve device and inhalation. The spacer device also reduces the velocity of the aerosol and allows more time for the medication to hang in the spacer until the patient is able to breathe it in, therefore depositing more of the medication in the lungs.

The mouthpiece should be wiped after each use with a damp cloth. Spacer devices should be cleaned with warm soapy water and left to 'air dry'. Drying with a cloth causes an electrostatic charge to accumulate on the interior surface of the spacer device which interferes with its performance, as the medication would then stick to the sides of the device rather than travelling down into the user's lungs. Spacer devices should be replaced every 6–12 months.

To use a large-volume spacer (Figure 9.2) you will first need to check that the inhaler device is compatible with the spacer. Instructions for use are given below.

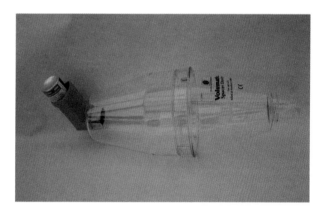

Figure 9.2 A large-volume spacer.

1   Fit the two halves of the spacer together.
2   Remove the mouthpiece of the inhaler and shake it well.
3   Fit the inhaler into one end of the spacer device, opposite the mouthpiece.
4   Ask the patient to place the mouthpiece into their mouth, making sure that the lips are sealed behind the ring.

5   Press the canister once and tell the patient to either breathe in and out slowly and deeply about four to six times, or breathe in slowly once and hold their breath for 10 seconds.

6   Ask the patient to remove the spacer from their mouth and then repeat the procedure for each dose of the drug. Wait one minute between each dose.

7   Do not put more than one dose of the drug into the spacer at any one time.

Prescriptions

All inhaled drugs must be used as per prescription for frequency and number of inhalations. Nebulised drugs are abbreviated as 'NEB' on the drug chart and inhalations are abbreviated as 'INH' on the chart.

Some individuals are instructed to take two inhalations. Others are told to wait a minute or two and take another inhalation only if necessary. Very often we see inhalers prescribed on the 'As Required' section of the prescription chart as *pro re nata* (PRN).

QUESTION

Question 9.1   What does PRN mean?

Common Mistakes in Inhaler Administration

* Not shaking the inhaler prior to use.
* Floating the inhaler in water to determine whether there is any medication left in the device.
* Not rinsing the mouth with water after administration.

Inhalers can cause oral thrush: look for white spots and furry tongue. This will require a prescription from a general practitioner (GP) to be rectified, for example nystatin.

How to Administer Medications with Inhaler Devices

Five of the most common inhaler devices you may see in the healthcare environment are the:

- Turbohaler,
- Metered-dose inhaler,
- Easi-Breathe,
- HandiHaler,
- Accuhaler.

Patients will be shown how to use the best device suitable for their needs by the respiratory specialists in the clinic, but may need to be reminded from time to time how to use and care for their device.

Turbohaler

The procedure for using a Turbohaler (Figure 9.3) is given below.

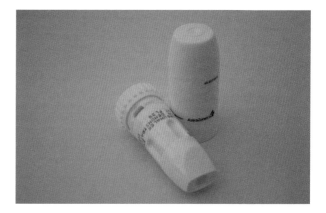

Figure 9.3 A Turbohaler inhaler.

1 Remove the lid by unscrewing from the inhaler.
2 Hold the Turbohaler upright and turn the bottom grip clockwise and then anticlockwise until it clicks.
3 Tell the patient to breathe out slowly and deeply to empty the lungs.

4   Now ask the patient place the mouthpiece between the
     lips and breathe in as quickly and as deeply as
     possible.

5   Tell the patient to hold their breath for as long as is
     comfortable (10 seconds).

To clean the Turbohaler wipe the mouthpiece with a dry
cloth or tissue.

Metered-Dose Inhaler

The procedure for using a metered-dose inhaler (Figure 9.4)
is given below.

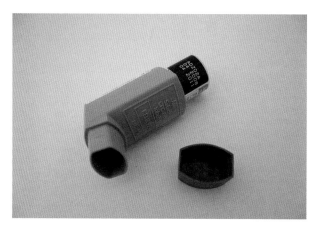

Figure 9.4 A metered-dose inhaler.

1   Remove the cap from the mouthpiece.
2   Shake the inhaler well.
3   Breathe out slowly.
4   Ask the patient to place the mouthpiece between the
     lips and start to breathe in slowly: tell them not to block
     the mouthpiece with the teeth or tongue. Press the
     canister *once* and tell them to continue breathing in as
     deeply and evenly as possible.
5   Tell them to hold their breathe for as long as is comfort-
     able (10 seconds).
6   Repeat the procedure after 30–60 seconds if another
     dose is needed.

To clean a metered-dose inhaler wipe the mouthpiece after use with a dry or damp cloth or tissue.

Easi-Breathe

The procedure for using an Easi-Breathe inhaler (Figure 9.5) is given below.

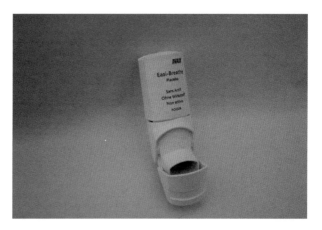

Figure 9.5 An Easi-Breathe inhaler.

1 Shake the inhaler.
2 Open the cap.
3 Tell the patient to breathe out slowly.
4 Have the patient place the mouthpiece firmly between the lips. Tell them to breathe in slowly and deeply through the mouthpiece but not to stop breathing in when the inhaler sends the dose into the mouth. They should continue to breathe in steadily after the dose is released until a deep breath has been taken. Care must be taken not to cover the air holes at the top of the device with the fingers.
5 Tell the patient to hold their breath for as long as is comfortable (10 seconds), and breathe out slowly.
6 Close the cap of the Easi-Breathe inhaler while holding the device in an upright position.
7 Repeat the procedure after at least one minute if a second dose is required.

To clean the Easi-Breathe inhaler wipe the mouthpiece after use with a dry or damp cloth or tissue.

HandiHaler

The procedure for using a HandiHaler (Figure 9.6) is given below.

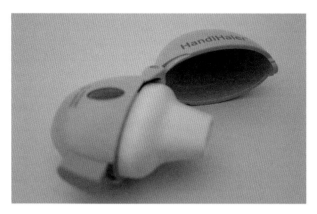

Figure 9.6 A HandiHaler inhaler. Source: Reproduced with permission.

1 Open the cap by pulling it upwards.
2 Pull open the mouthpiece.
3 Remove the medication capsule from the blister pack and place it in the centre chamber.
4 Close the mouthpiece firmly until a click is heard, leaving the cap open.
5 Tell the patient to hold the HandiHaler with the mouthpiece upwards and press the green button once, and release.
6 Ask the patient to breathe out completely.
7 Ask the patient to place the HandiHaler in their mouth and close their lips tightly around the mouthpiece.
8 The patient should keep the head in an upright position and breathe in slowly and deeply until they hear the capsule vibrate.
9 They should then breathe in until their lungs are full, and then hold their breath for as long as is comfortable (10 seconds).

10   Tell them to breathe out slowly.

11   Repeat steps 5 and 6 to ensure that the capsule has been emptied completely.

12   Open the mouthpiece again and tip out the used capsule.

13   Close the mouthpiece and replace the cap.

To clean the HandiHaler open the cap and mouthpiece. Open the base by lifting the piercing button. Rinse the HandiHaler thoroughly with warm water to remove any powder. Dry the HandiHaler thoroughly by tipping excess water out onto a paper towel. Leave the inhaler to dry naturally in the open air. These devices take approximately 24 hours to dry. The mouthpiece may be cleaned between uses with a dry cloth.

Accuhaler

The procedure for using a Accuhaler (Figure 9.7) is given below.

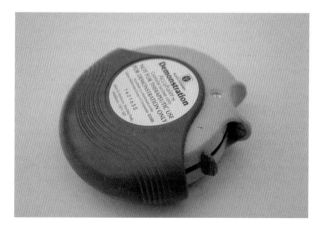

Figure 9.7 An Accuhaler inhaler. Source: Reproduced with permission.

1   To open the Accuhaler, hold the outer case in one hand, place the thumb of your other hand on the thumb grip and push away from you until you hear a click.

2   Tell the patient to hold the Accuhaler level, with the mouthpiece facing them. Then slide the lever on the side of the device away from you until you hear it click. Each time the lever is pushed back a new blister is prepared for breathing in and this is shown on the dose counter. The lever should only be pressed when the medication is required.

3   Tell the patient to breathe out gently away from the inhaler. They should close their lips firmly around the mouthpiece and breathe in steadily and deeply through the Accuhaler.

4   Then they should hold their breath for as long as is comfortable (10 seconds), and breathe out slowly.

5   Close the Accuhaler by placing your thumb in the thumb grip and sliding it back towards you until you hear it click shut. If a second blister is to be inhaled, repeat the procedure.

To clean the Accuhaler wipe the mouthpiece with a dry tissue.

Other Treatments for asthma

For individuals with severe asthma, other interventions may be required to relieve their symptoms:

Tablets – such as steroid tablets, Theophylline tablets/capsules, Leukotriene receptor antagonist (LTRAs) which also come in syrup and powder form

Injections – Benralizumab (Fasenra), Omalizumab (Xolair), Mepolizumab (Nucala), Reslizumab (Cinqaero)

Surgery – A procedure called a bronchial thermoplasty may be offered as a treatment for severe asthma.

TEST YOUR KNOWLEDGE

1   A patient has just been prescribed salbutamol to be delivered by a metered-dose inhaler. They seem very distressed and state they can't remember how to take it. Talk the patient through the procedure and care advice.

KEY POINTS

- The principles of administering medications via nebulisation and aerosolisation.
- Looking at the medical conditions of asthma and COPD and medication and devices used in these conditions.

WEB RESOURCES

BNF Adults: www.bnf.nice.org.uk
BNF Children: www.bnfc.nice.org.uk
The Royal Marsden Clinical Nursing Procedures:
  www.rmmonline.co.uk/manual
You will need to register and log in.
Asthma: www.asthma.org.uk
www.nhs.uk/conditions/asthma/treatment

Chapter 10
· ·
ADMINISTRATION OF INTRAVENOUS FLUIDS

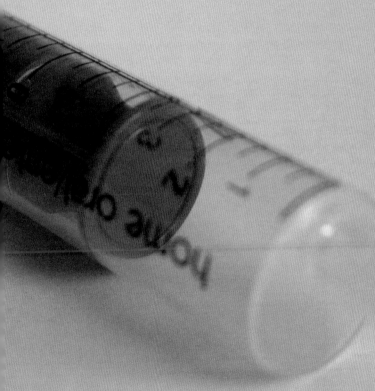

Medicine Management Skills for Nurses, Second Edition. Claire Boyd.
© 2022 John Wiley & Sons Ltd. Published 2022 by John Wiley & Sons Ltd.

When administering medications via the intravenous (or IV)
route, the patient must have a patent peripheral venous
cannula sited in a vein. Peripheral venous cannulation is
when a plastic or metal tube is inserted into a peripheral
vein so that the patient can receive intravenous therapy,
such as IV fluids and/or drugs, or transfusion of blood
products. A further indication of use is the administration of
dyes and contrast media during clinical investigations.

You may also hear a peripheral venous cannula being called
a peripheral venous catheter, or PVC, and it is often
commonly referred to simply as a cannula. Another name for
it is venflon.

As the cannula sits in the vein, medications transfused into it
will be administered via the IV route. The patient in
Figure 10.1 is having an IV infusion set up.

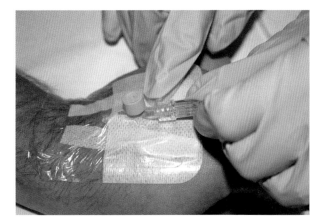

Figure 10.1 A patient having an IV infusion set up,
through a cannula.

IV fluids are administered over a set time, for example eight hours. Infusions that take more than over 5 minutes but less than 24 hours to administer are known as **intermittent intravenous infusions**. Anything administered over 24 hours is referred to as a **continuous infusion,** for example, insulin or heparin.

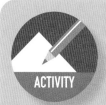

Activity 10.1

ACTIVITY

Why do you think drugs are administered via the IV route (as IV fluids, injections and by continuous infusion)? List as many reasons as you can.

TYPES OF FLUID REPLACEMENT

One of the reasons why IV drugs are delivered is that a patient requires *rapid fluid replacement*. The types of fluid we would use include:

* crystalloids, such as normal saline (NaCl), 5% dextrose,
* colloids, such as Gelofusine or Haemaccel,
* blood, such as concentrated red blood cells (or RBCs).

Crystalloids

Crystalloids are categorised according to their osmolarity compared with plasma osmolarity (osmolarity is explained below). There are three types:

* isotonic, which has the *same* osmolarity as plasma;
* hypotonic, which has a *lower* osmolarity than plasma;
* hypertonic, which has a *higher* osmolarity than plasma.

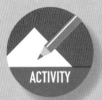

Activity 10.2

Can you think of one example for each of these?

1   Isotonic
2   Hypotonic
3   Hypertonic

Blood Products are Hypertonic

Crystalloids and colloids are both isotonic effective volume expanders for short periods of time only. This means they are good to administer to hypotensive and hypovolaemic patients.

Figure 10.2 shows a list of some of the IV fluids used in clinical practice

0.9% Sodium Chloride	Fluid of choice for routine maintenance. Suitable for use in resuscitation in hypovolaemic shock.
0.9% Sodium Chloride + 5% Dextrose	Suitable for maintenance fluid therapy in infants and children requiring isotonic fluid and for patients with hypoglycaemia.
0.45% Sodium Chloride + 5% Dextrose	Suitable for maintenance fluid therapy in infants and children.
0.45% Sodium Chloride + 10% Dextrose	Suitable for maintenance fluid therapy in infants and children with hypoglycaemia
Hartmann's solution	Can be used for intra-operative and post-operative use.
10% Dextrose in water	May be used to treat hypoglycaemia

Figure 10.2 IV Fluids.

Osmolarity

You won't be surprised to hear that *osmolarity* is connected with *osmosis*. This is the movement of water through a selectively permeable membrane. Pores in the membrane allow the water molecules to move back and forth, but the direction of movement will be from a high water concentration to a low water concentration, meaning the water moves from a weak solution to a stronger, more concentrated, solution.

Our cells have a selectively permeable membrane and if we put some of our cells into a beaker of fluid with the same concentration as our body fluid (known as *isotonic*) there would be no movement of fluids either into or out of the cells.

If we put our cells into a beaker of fluid with a higher concentration than our body fluids (known as *hypertonic*), the cells would shrink as the fluid leaves the cells and enters the fluid in the beaker.

If we put our cells into a beaker of fluid with a lower concentration than our body fluid (known as *hypotonic*) the cells would swell and burst as they drew in the fluid from the solution.

In healthy adults, the body consists of approximately 50–65% water. Babies have approximately 70%. Older people have less. This water is located around the body in intracellular and extracellular compartments. Most of the water is actually within the cells: the intracellular fluid (ICF). Extracellular fluid (ECF) is tissue fluid that bathes the cells and blood plasma, consisting of *interstitial fluid*. Other types of ECF are lymph, gastrointestinal juices, and the cerebro-spinal fluid around the brain and spinal cord.

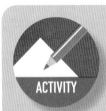

Activity 10.3

What is it called when we have an excess of water in the interstitial fluid? How is it recognised?

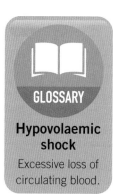

Hypovolaemic shock

Excessive loss of circulating blood.

DEHYDRATION

Dehydration occurs when excess fluid is lost from the body (or inadequate amounts have been taken in). Water is lost from the extracellular fluid and fluid then moves out of the cells to equalise the concentration of the intracellular and extracellular fluids.

Dehydration can be caused due to conditions such as diarrhoea, vomiting, severe sweating, severe burns and scalds, diabetes mellitus, and hypovolaemic shock, when a large amount of blood loss has occurred.

The aim with a dehydrated patient is to rehydrate the individual orally, via a naso-gastric tube, intravenously, or by subcutaneous infusion. Patients may also lose electrolytes during severe episodes of diarrhoea and vomiting. Electrolytes are positively and negatively charged ions in the ICF and ECF compartments.

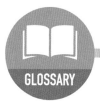

Electrolyte

A solution that produces ions; for example, sodium chloride solution consists of free sodium and free chloride ions.

The ion concentrations in these compartments can be seen in Table 10.1.

Table 10.1 Intracellular and extracellular fluids.

Intracellular fluid contains. . .	Extracellular fluid contains
Large qualities of organic phosphates and proteins	Large quantities of hydrogen carbonate and chloride in interstitial fluid Large quantities of these ions and protein in plasma
Small quantities of hydrogen carbonate (bicarbonate) and chloride	Small quantities of hydrogen phosphate, sulphate, and organic ions
Large quantities of potassium and magnesium	Large quantities of sodium
Small quantities of sodium	Small quantities of potassium, magnesium, and calcium

A common investigation in health care is to investigate the serum electrolytes in the blood. The results of these levels can guide us in determining our patient's health status. Common results are found in Table 10.2 but may vary slightly in clinical areas.

Table 10.2 Electrolyte ranges.

Electrolyte	Normal range (mmol/l)
Sodium	135–145
Chloride	95–105
Potassium	3.3–5.0
Hydrogen carbonate (bicarbonate)	22–30
Calcium	2.12–2.65
Magnesium	0.75–1.5

RISK TO THE PATIENT

Administering medications via the intravenous route, through a cannula, can present risks to the patient. We need to be vigilant of:

- over-infusion; for example congestive cardiac failure (CCF) or electrolyte imbalance,
- under-infusion; for example dehydration/electrolyte imbalance,
- infiltration: inadvertently administering the drug into surrounding tissues (may cause tissue damage and/or oedema),
- extravasation: inadvertently administering a vesicant substance into the tissues, causing extended tissue damage,
- cellulitis: intravenous-related infection. Asepsis should be maintained at insertion, during clinical use and at removal of the cannula.
- phlebitis: inflammation of the vein (regular monitoring of the intravenous access site is important),
- systemic complications: including sepsis, pulmonary thromboembolism, air embolism, and catheter-fragment embolism,
- anaphylactic/allergic reaction,

- inability to recall (that is, remove) the drug and reverse its action,
- thrombus (blood clot): air entering the cardiovascular system. A mechanical thrombus occurs when a broken piece of cannula or glass from an ampoule, or rubber from ampoule, enters the vein.

GLOSSARY

Vesicant

An infused IV fluid that enters the extravascular space and causes irritation to the vein, resulting in blistering, tissue injury, and/or necrosis.

COMPLICATIONS OF IV THERAPY

Administering large volumes of IV fluids can potentially be very dangerous in certain patients, as can the speed at which they receive their medication, and certain factors should be considered, such as:

- If the patient is at risk, such as cardiac failure, avoid free flow by using a pump.
- If using a gravity feed, remember your drip-rate formula (see Chapter 4).
- Observe all infusions frequently.
- Patients receiving their intravenous infusion without a pump must be monitored closely.
- Beware of the cannula being 'positional'; that is, improperly sited in the vein and prone to being dislodged.
- Confused patients or relatives may open a clamp or valve to make an infusion to go through quicker, with the potential for free flow and speed shock.
- Perform accurate vital sign monitoring.
- Beware of speed shock.
- Remember that the composition, viscosity, and concentration of a fluid can affect its flow.

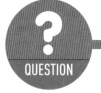

QUESTION

Question 10.1   What are free flow and speed shock?

For gravity-fed infusions – meaning an infusion that is not put through a pump – you should allow approximately 1 m from the patient's shoulder to the fluid being infused. This provides 70 mmHg of pressure which is adequate to overcome venous pressure (the normal range in adults is 25–80 mmHg).

As our patient alternates their position, such as by standing up or lying down from a sitting position, the flow rate will change and a re-counting of the drip rate will be required.

ADDING MEDICATIONS TO BAGS OF FLUID

When adding drugs to a bag of fluids you will need to mix well. This is performed by inverting the bag several times and not shaking. Figure 10.3 shows how the medication can fall to the bottom of the bag and then be administered in far too concentrated a dose. Mixing well at the start means that the medication is distributed within the bag and does not drop down like this (known as precipitation) if given within the correct time frame: isn't science wonderful!

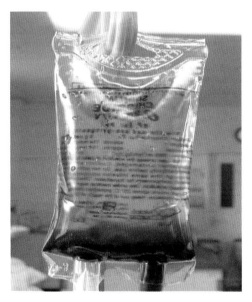

Figure 10.3 Medication may fall to the bottom of a bag and become too concentrated.

EQUIPMENT

In order to administer an intravenous infusion, you will require an administration set (see below), often referred to as a 'giving set'. You will also require the medication to be infused, a drip stand (Figure 10.4), personal protective equipment (gloves and apron), and a sterile swab to wipe the cannula.

A clear-fluid administration set (Figure 10.5) delivers 20 drops/ml. It is in the clear chamber (shown in the picture) that we count the drip rate: that is, how many drops drip down into this chamber per minute. This type of administration set needs to be changed every 72 hours.

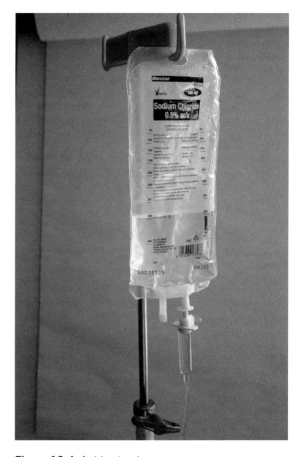

Figure 10.4 A drip stand.

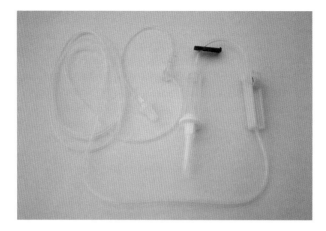

Figure 10.5 A clear- or thin-fluid administration line.

BLOOD PRODUCTS

A bag of blood is usually administered over three to four hours and with an administration set (Figure 10.6) that delivers 15 drops/ml. These sets have filters. Blood products should ideally be delivered through a pump. This type of administration set needs to be changed every 12 hours.

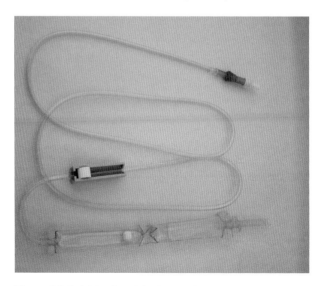

Figure 10.6 A blood and thickened-fluid administration line.

INFUSION DEVICES

Infusion devices (Figure 10.7) used to deliver IV fluids are called volumetric infusion pumps, or syringe drivers, and there are many on the market. You will be trained in how to use these pumps and assessed for competency. Many pumps deliver fluids in millilitres per hour and work this out for you, but the formula we can use to check this is:

$$\text{Infusion rate} = \frac{\text{amount of fluid}\,(\text{mL})}{\text{infusion time}\,(\text{hours})}$$

Chapter 4 looks at how to calculate the rates of Infusions in more detail.

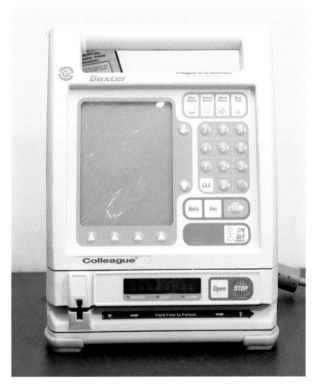

Figure 10.7 An infusion device (Lister, Hofner, and Graton 2020).

Calculating the Drip Rate

This calculation is required for gravity-fed Infusions (the manual method for working out the infusion rate) and gives us an answer in drops per minute. In order to calculate the rate, in drops per minute, the following formula is used:

$$\text{Rate} = \frac{\text{volume}}{\text{time in hours}} \times \frac{\text{drops per millilitre}}{\text{minutes per hour}}$$

Again, Chapter 6 looks at this in more detail.

PRESCRIPTIONS

All IV fluids, whether glucose, sodium chloride, or blood products, have to be prescribed. A typical prescription for intravenous fluid will look something like Figure 10.8.

Date	Intravenous Fluid	Volume	Duration	Additive and Dose	Prescriber's Signature	Batch Number	Nurse's Signature	Time Started	Time Completed
Today	0.9% Sodium chloride	1 litre	6 hours	None	A. Medic				

Figure 10.8 Part of a prescription chart for intravenous fluid.

A fluid chart will need to be commenced, if one has not already been started.

A typical prescription form for a blood product can be seen In Figure 10.9. Sections 1, 2, 3, and 4 will be completed. It is this form you will take with you to collect the blood from the fridge in the blood lab.

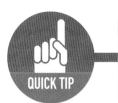

QUICK TIP

On a fluid chart a patient's fluid input (drinks, IV medications, etc.) and fluid output (urine, diarrhoea, vomit, wound drains) are recorded, allowing you to establish the fluid balance, or the input minus the output.

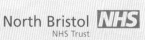

North Bristol **NHS**
NHS Trust

BLOOD TRANSFUSION RECORD

It is Trust policy to complete as a minimum:
Section 1: Indication for Transfusion   Section 3: Agreement to Transfusion   Section 4: Prescription
Section 5: Blood Collection   Record of Administration: to record date, time & staff signatures

Hospital..
Ward/Dept...
Directorate...
Consultant...

Affix patient addressograph here or complete below:

Surname: ....
First Name(s): ....
Hospital No: .... **DOB** ....

1.   Indication for Transfusion

An Hb threshold of **7g/dl** in otherwise fit patients (8g/dl in older patients and those with known / likely cardiovascular disease) is recommended unless symptomatic or active bleeding.
Transfusion to an Hb above 10g/dl is very rarely indicated unless patient is red cell dependent or a neonate.
Symptoms / signs ....
Diagnosis causing low Hb / anaemia / bleeding...

2.   Relevant Medical History   Special considerations.................................

Pre-transfusion Haemoglobin ....g/dl   Blood group ....
Previous transfusion / blood product Yes / No   Previous reaction:Yes / No When: ....
If yes, what and when? ....

3.   Agreement to Transfusion

This patient has verbally agreed to a blood transfusion and has received relevant information leaflets or
this patient has <u>not</u> provided consent because..
Date .... Staff signature.................................... Print name ....

4.   Prescription

Sections 1, 2 and 3 should be completed with prescription, except when 2 & 3 can be done pre-operation
N.B During surgery, prescription on an anaesthetic record is an acceptable alternative

Product & Amount	Date for infusion	Special requirements	Rate	Dr name, sign, date & time

5.   Blood Collection (Take blood transfusion record to fridge) *(Requestor & Receiver please sign, and record date & time)*

		Unit 1	Unit 2	Unit 3	Unit 4	Unit 5	Unit 6
Requestor: check patient ID at bedside, patient ID confirmed with collector	Sign Date Time						
Receiver: take receipt of blood	Sign: Date Time						

Figure 10.9 Prescription form for a blood product. Source: Permission to reproduce this image is granted by North Bristol NHS Trust and University Hospitals Bristol NHS Foundation Trust.

PREPARATION OF INTRAVENOUS FLUIDS

1 Collect all equipment.

2 *Wash your hands.*

3 Two checkers are required for IV therapy.

4 Apply aseptic principles.

5 Check that you have the correct patient and obtain consent.

6 Inspect the fluid bag to be certain that it contains the correct fluid, the fluid is clear (if the medication should be), the bag is not leaking and the bag has not expired.

7 Sterile packaging must not be damaged or wet.

8 Ensure that you have the correct giving set for the fluid to be administered. This can be either a microdrip set – which delivers 60 drops/ml into the drip chamber – or a macrodrip set – which delivers 15–20 drops/ml into the drip chamber.

9 Open the packaging and uncoil the tubing: do not let the ends of the tubing become contaminated. Close the flow regulator (roll the wheel away from the end you will attach the fluid bag to).

10 Remove the protective covering from the port of the fluid bag and the protective covering from the spike of the administration set.

11 Insert the spike of the administration set into the port of the fluid bag with a quick twist. Do this carefully. Be especially careful not to puncture yourself! Insert this spike fully into the infusion bag, as this is an infection risk.

12 Hold the fluid bag higher than the drip chamber of the administration set. Squeeze the drip chamber once or twice to start the flow. Fill the drip chamber to one-third full. If you overfill the chamber, lower the bag below the level of the drip chamber and squeeze some fluid back into the fluid bag.

13 Open the flow regulator and allow the fluid to flush all the air from the tubing. Let it run into the giving set's empty packaging or container. You may need to loosen or remove the cap at the end of the tubing to

get the fluid to flow to the end of the tubing (but this should not be necessary), taking care not to let the tip of the administration set become contaminated.

14 The primed giving set is now ready to be connected to an electronic device, or the rate can be determined by gravity flow together with the flow clamp.

15 Connect the end of the tubing to the patient: the intravenous cannula must be of an appropriate size for the intended use and cleaned with an alcohol swab or similar, such as a Clinell Wipe. Leave the cannula to dry before the giving-set end is attached, to minimize infection risk.

PROCEDURE FOR DISCONNECTION OF INTRAVENOUS INFUSION

1 On completion of infusion, switch off the volumetric infusion pump – if using – and clamp the infusion set tubing, removing it from the pump.

2 Wash your hands and apply a gloves and apron.

3 Using aseptic technique disconnect from the peripheral cannula. Insert a new sterile peripheral bung.

4 A registered nurse, midwife, or assistant practitioner must flush the peripheral cannula with 0.9% sodium chloride to maintain patency.

5 Check the peripheral cannula site and record details.

6 Replace dressing or remove cannula if required.

7 Correctly dispose of equipment into a clinical waste bag and suitable sharps container.

8 Clean and return the infusion stand and volumetric pump to the designated storage area.

9 Wash your hands.

TEST YOUR KNOWLEDGE

1 Are blood products isotonic, hypotonic, or hypertonic?

2 How often should an IV administration set be changed when delivering clear fluids?

3 How often should a filtered IV administration set be changed when delivering blood products?

4   500 ml of normal saline is going through an infusion device over four hours. What is the rate in millilitres per hour?

5   1 l of normal saline is prescribed to go through over eight hours. There is no infusion device available. What is the drip rate in drops per minute?

6   400 ml of blood is to be transfused over three hours. What is the rate in drops per min? No infusion device is available.

KEY POINTS

- The types of IV fluid replacement.
- Complications associated with the administration of IV therapy.
- Documents associated with IV fluids, including blood transfusion records.
- The procedure for administering IV fluids.

WEB RESOURCES

BNF Adults: www.bnf.nice.org.uk
BNF Children: www.bnfc.nice.org.uk

REFERENCE

Lister, S., Hofland, J., and Graton, Hayley (eds.). (2020). *The Royal Marsden of Clinical Nursing Procedures*, 10e. Wiley.

Chapter 11

* *

ADMINISTRATION OF INTRAVENOUS BOLUS MEDICATIONS

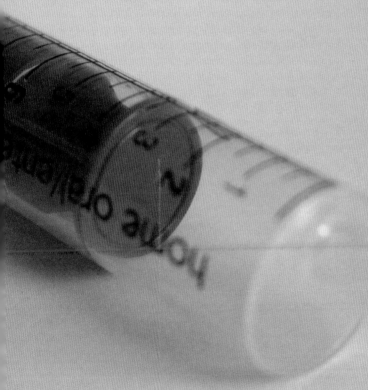

Medicine Management Skills for Nurses, Second Edition. Claire Boyd.
© 2022 John Wiley & Sons Ltd. Published 2022 by John Wiley & Sons Ltd.

LEARNING OUTCOMES

By the end of this chapter you will have an understanding of the theory and practice of the clinical skill of administering intravenous (IV) bolus medications.

Bolus injections, also known as IV push or direct intermittent injection, are small volumes of medication solutions delivered through a peripheral vascular access device, otherwise known as a cannula into the vein.

A bolus injection may need to be administered over 3–10 minutes, depending on the drug. For instance, furosemide (administered for oedema) should be administered at a rate not usually exceeding 4 mg/min or tinnitus and deafness may result due to speed shock. Bolus injections are also administered to minimise vein irritation and the risk of extravasation. This includes drugs such as penicillin antibiotics (e.g. amoxicillin) and antiemetics (e.g. cyclizine).

During emergency situations, a bolus injection can be given at a much quicker rate due to the clinical need outweighing the risk of speed shock and extravasation. For example, if a patient is experiencing cardiac arrhythmias, adenosine needs to reach the heart as soon as possible for immediate effect.

ADVANTAGES OF IV BOLUS INJECTIONS

- Achieves immediate effect.
- Delivers high medicine levels.
- Easier to prepare for the practitioner than an infusion: no setting-up of infusion devices.
- After administering the dose, the practitioner does not need to monitor an infusion device, as they would with continuous infusion.

SALINE FLUSHES

Saline flushes are administered to keep the cannula patent. When administering IV flushes through a cannula, a 'push pause' method is used. This means that we stop and start the administration of the fluid – for example 1 ml in, wait a moment, 1 ml in, wait a moment – until all the flush has been used. This push pause method is used to create lots of episodes of turbulence, which removes any small particles of debris that have built up at the end of the cannula.

DISADVANTAGES OF IV BOLUS INJECTIONS

* Increased potential for adverse effects, especially if drug administered too quickly; for example, furosemide.
* Potential to cause damage to the veins; for example, phlebitis or extravasation.

Let me show you an example. . . with amoxicillin

Let's put all this information into practice and let me show you how I would go about administering a bolus injection of amoxicillin.

NOTE: clinical areas may vary slightly in the administration of this drug, so always check first.

Look at the prescription chart (Figure 11.1). A doctor has prescribed amoxicillin to my adult patient, who I know has pneumonia. The first thing I do is check the prescription in the *British National Formulary* (BNF): has the medic got the dose right? Yes, I am quite happy that 500 mg of amoxicillin is correct, and can be given every eight hours. In children up to 10 years of age the dose is 250 mg every eight hours, but it can be doubled in a severe infection.

6 hourly	06.00 – 12.00 – 18.00 – 23.00	SURNAME (MR/MRS/MISS)		DATE OF BIRTH	UNIT NUMBER
8 hourly	06.00 – 14.00 – 22.00	FIRST NAMES		SEX	CONSULTANT
12 hourly	09.00 – 21.00	ADDRESS			

REGULAR PRESCRIPTIONS

	Date	Drug (approved name – BLOCK CAPITALS)	Dose	Route	Times of Administration 6	14	,		22	Other Directions/ Duration	Doctor's Signature	Date	Pharm
1	TODAY	Amoxicillin	500MG	IV	√	√			√	7 Days then STOP	A Doctor		
2													
3													
4													
5													

Figure 11.1 The patient's prescription chart, completed by a doctor.
Source: Permission to reproduce this image is granted by North Bristol NHS Trust and University Hospitals Bristol NHS Foundation Trust.

I will need to confirm that my patient does not have an allergy or sensitivity to penicillin. I will also need to check that the doctor has written in a stop date for the penicillin. The doctor has written that the drug is to be given by the IV route, but does not state whether this is to be added to a bag of fluid and delivered through a volumetric pump, or in a syringe and delivered through a syringe driver, or to be given by bolus injection. This means that, if the medication can be given in these forms, the choice is mine. I check and find that amoxicillin can be given in the following ways.

Adults and Children

- Intermittent bolus injection: added to water for injection (WFI) and given over three to four minutes.
- IV infusion: added to solution and given over 30–60 minutes.
- Intramuscular (IM) injection: added to WFI (Table 11.1, p. 183).

Neonates

- IV infusion via syringe pump: added to solution and given over 30 minutes.

Table 11.1 Dilution and rates for administering amoxicillin.

Method	Dilution	Rate (min)
IV bolus (preferred method)	If using a whole vial: add 5 ml WFI to 250 mg vial or 10 ml WFI to 500 mg vial. If using part of a vial: add 4.8 ml to 250 mg vial or 9.6 ml to 500 mg vial. This gives a 50 mg/ml solution.	Over 3–4
IV infusion	Reconstitute the vial as above. Add the solution to 50–250 ml of normal saline (NS), glucose (G), or glucose saline (GS).	Over 30–60

Next I check that we have the medication in the stock cupboard and how it is presented. I find that we keep 250 and 500 mg vials. Now I check the method, dilution, and rate (Table 11.2).

Did you notice in the table that IV bolus is the preferred method? But if using this option, I need to administer it over a three to four minute time span. I need to check at this point that my patient has a patent cannula in place.

Before I wash my hands, put on an apron and gloves and gather all my equipment, I need to read and be aware of any further information I will require when administering this drug. I find out:

- Infusion-related adverse events: nausea, vomiting, hypersensitivity reactions including rash, fever, joint pain, and angioedema,
- pH 8–10 (after reconstitution with WFI),
- Flush: normal saline (NS; 0.9% sodium chloride),
- Displacement value: 250 mg vial = 0.2 ml; 500 mg vial = 0.4 ml.

We will look at displacement value a little later on, but the infusion-related adverse reactions need to be explained to my patient before they consent to having this medication; they should let me know immediately if they start to feel unwell.

After the patient has consented, and I wash my hands, put on my apron and gather the drug, needles, a sharps bin, and clean injection tray, my flush, syringes, and cleaning swab, I start to prepare everything. I ask a colleague to check the prescription chart with me and the medication dates, dose, and route.

I draw up 10 ml WFI in a 20 ml syringe and add some of this to the amoxicillin vial and mix well. I do not remove the needle and syringe. I then draw the contents of the vial back into the syringe and change the needle and invert this syringe to mix the contents well. I change needles. Best practice, is to label this medication so that I do not confuse the drug with the flush. Then I draw up the NS flush, usually 5–10 ml.

I then go to the patient and check all the details:

right medicine is given,
to the **right patient**,
at the **right time**,
in the **right form**,
at the **right dose**.

I clean the hub of the cannula and allow this to dry. I check the cannula site for any visible signs of phlebitis. I then add half of the NS flush, asking the patient if they feel any pain. If the patient complains of pain, I will immediately stop. This will mean that a new cannula will need to be inserted and the troublesome one removed. If the cannula is fine to use, I administer the amoxicillin over three to four minutes, then finish with the rest of the NS flush. I immediately put the used syringes and needles into the sharps bin and sign the prescription chart. I dispose of all equipment and wash my hands.

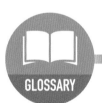
GLOSSARY

Phlebitis
Inflammation of a vein.

Chemical phlebitis
Irritation to a vein instigated by drug therapy.

Mechanical phlebitis
Irritation to a vein caused by movement of a cannula.

Bacterial phlebitis
Inflammation of a vein caused by bacterial infection.

AMOXICILLIN ADMINISTRATION IN NEONATES

My IV drug administration instruction book tells me that when administering amoxicillin to neonates it is best to deliver the drug through a syringe pump. The instructions are given in Table 11.2.

Table 11.2 Instructions for administering amoxicillin to a neonate.

Method	Dilution	Rate (min)
IV infusion via a syringe pump	Add 4.8 ml to a 250 mg vial or 9.6 ml to a 500 mg vial. This gives a 50 mg/ml solution	Over 30

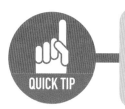

QUICK TIP

But I thought we had to add 5 ml of WFI to a 250 mg vial?

No, we add 4.8 ml, which will give us 5 ml. This is due to displacement: let me explain.

DISPLACEMENT

Some drugs, especially antibiotics, are freeze-dried (Figure 11.2). They are presented in solid form in the vial and need to be reconstituted with a known volume of solution before they can be administered.

These powders can displace a certain amount of fluid, known as the **displacement value** of the drug, and this must be taken into account when only part of the vial is being used. If this is not done, serious errors in dosage can occur and this is especially dangerous when working out paediatric doses, and those in critical care.

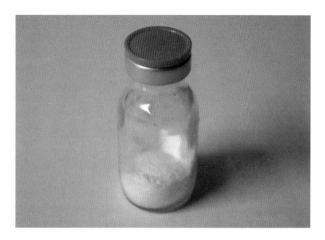

Figure 11.2 A freeze-dried drug.

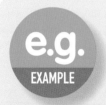

Let me show you an example. . .

Adjusting the liquid amount at the start:

- To give a dose of 125 mg amoxicillin from a 250 mg vial the WFI is 5 ml, but we must take into account the displacement value for amoxicillin, which for 250 mg is 0.2 ml.
- So, adding 4.8 ml of fluid will give a total of 5 ml in the vial, and therefore 250 mg in 5 ml.
- To administer 125 mg, you will need to administer 2.5 ml of the solution.

So, can you see you don't actually add 5 ml of WFI to the vial but 5–0.2 = 4.8 ml. This will then make up 5 ml in our syringe as the powder, once dissolved, contributes to the volume.

SPEED SHOCK

Speed shock is described as being the rapid uncontrolled administration of a drug, where symptoms occur as a result of the speed with which medication is administered rather than the volume of drug or fluid. This can therefore occur even with small volumes. An example of this is a drug called furosemide, which is administered for oedema. If given too fast it can cause the patient to experience tinnitus or permanent deafness.

This drug has to be administered at a rate of 4 mg/min (remember this information at the start of this chapter – who was paying attention?!).

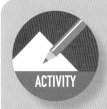

Activity 11.1

A child has been prescribed 20 mg of furosemide daily. Over what time period should this bolus injection be administered?

Infiltration V Extravasation

IV drugs need to be administered via a peripheral access device, such as a cannula to get the medication into the vein, but if this cannula dislodges from the vein and the infused non-vesicant substance enters the surrounding tissue – infiltration occurs. We used to call this 'tissuing'. You will notice swelling around the cannula area and patient may complain of pain on administration of the IV drug. If the substance being infused is a vesicant (which means blister forming, as described in Chapter 10), and the substance enters the tissues, more tissue damage may be caused, including tissue death.

DNA binding vesicants, such as doxorubicin, bind to nucleic acids in the DNA of healthy cells, resulting in cell death, whereas non-DNA binding vesicants, such as Vinca alkaloids, have an indirect rather than direct effect on the cells.

DID YOU KNOW?

Vinca alkaloids are a class of anti-cancer drugs derived from the Madagasca periwinkle plant.

If extravasation is evident, the person administering the medication must know the group of drug that has caused the problem due to the fact that drugs from Group A and drugs from Group B have different antidotes.

GROUP A DRUGS

Vinca Alkaloids (Vinblastine, Vindesine, Vinorelbine, Vincristine, Vinflunine)
Paclitaxel
Calcium chloride
Calcium gluconate

Phenytoin
Hypertonic solutions, such as:
    Sodium chloride > 0.9%
    Sodium bicarbonate > 5%
    Glucose 50%

GROUP B DRUGS

Amsacrine
Concentrated Carmustine
Concentrated Dacarbazine
Dactinomycin
Daunorubicin
Doxorubicin
Epirubicin
Idarubicin
Amrubicin
Actinomycin D
Mitomycin C
Mechlorethamine

Streptozocin
Aciclovir
Amphotericin
Cefotaxime
Diazepam
Ganciclovir
Mannitol
Potassium chloride > 40 mmol/l
Potassium phosphate
Thiopental

Managing Extravasation

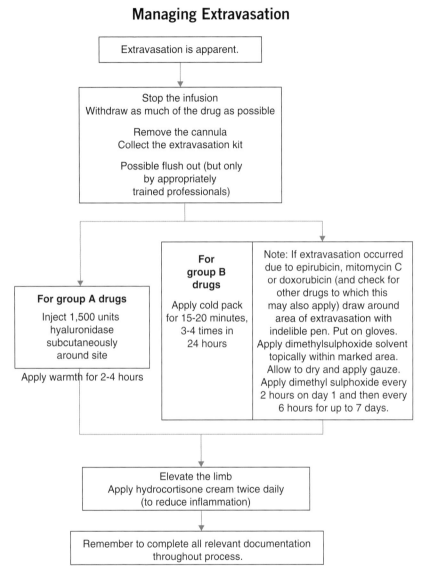

Extravasation is apparent.

Stop the infusion
Withdraw as much of the drug as possible

Remove the cannula
Collect the extravasation kit

Possible flush out (but only
by appropriately
trained professionals)

For group A drugs

Inject 1,500 units
hyaluronidase
subcutaneously
around site

Apply warmth for 2-4 hours

**For
group B
drugs**

Apply cold pack
for 15-20 minutes,
3-4 times in
24 hours

Note: If extravasation occurred
due to epirubicin, mitomycin C
or doxorubicin (and check for
other drugs to which this
may also apply) draw around
area of extravasation with
indelible pen. Put on gloves.
Apply dimethylsulphoxide solvent
topically within marked area.
Allow to dry and apply gauze.
Apply dimethyl sulphoxide every
2 hours on day 1 and then every
6 hours for up to 7 days.

Elevate the limb
Apply hydrocortisone cream twice daily
(to reduce inflammation)

Remember to complete all relevant documentation
throughout process.

Solutions with a high or low pH have the potential to cause
more tissue damage if they are extravasated.

DID YOU KNOW

The drug Phenytoin has the same pH as bleach!

Remember, the pH of blood is 7.35–7.45. Below are some examples of medicine pH levels, Figure 11.3.

Aciclovir	pH 11
Adrenaline	pH 2.5–3.6
Allopurinol	pH 10.8–11.8
Amiodarone	pH 3.5–4.5
Cyclizine	pH 3.3–3.7
Furosemide	pH 8–9.5
Morphine	pH 3–6
Omeprazole	pH 9–10
Phenytoin Sodium	pH 12
Quinine Dihydrochloride	pH 1.5–3
Salbutamol	pH 3–5
Vancomycin	pH 2.8–4.5
Fentanyl	pH 4–7.5
Tetracycline	pH 1–8

Figure 11.3 The pH of medicines.

DID YOU KNOW

The term pH stands for potential hydrogen. It describes the acidity or basicity of a solution. The pH scale ranges from 0 to 14 with 0 being the most acid, e.g. hydrochloric acid and 14 being the most alkaline, e.g. sodium hydroxide.

TEST YOUR KNOWLEDGE

Displacement: a patient is prescribed 1.5 g ceftazidime BD (twice daily), administered as a bolus. You have been provided with a 2 g vial, which needs to be reconstituted (with WFI) to make a total volume of 10 ml.

1   How many millilitres of this solution will you draw up to administer 1.5 g? Displacement value is 1.5 ml/2 g vial.
2   What volume of the drug do you need to draw up to administer 1.5 g of the drug?
3   What is the pH of blood?
4   What is the pH of the anti-emetic cyclizine?

KEY POINTS

- The principles of administering bolus injections.
- How to account for displacement values when reconstituting drugs.
- How to administer IV amoxicillin to neonates.
- The dangers of speed shock.
- Managing extravasation
- The pH of certain medications

WEB RESOURCES

BNF: www.bnf.nice.org.uk
Pharmacy: www.rpharms.com
Electronic Medicines Compendium: www.medicines.org.uk/emc

REFERENCE

Dougherty, L. and Lister, S. (eds.) (2011). *Royal Marsden Manual of Clinical Nursing Procedures*, 9e. Wiley.

Chapter 12
· · · · · · · · · · · · · · · · · · · ·
ADMINISTRATION OF CONTINUOUS INTRAVENOUS INFUSIONS

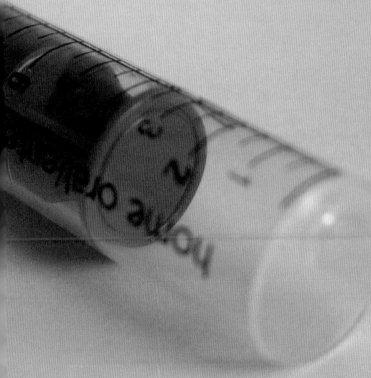

Medicine Management Skills for Nurses, Second Edition. Claire Boyd.
© 2022 John Wiley & Sons Ltd. Published 2022 by John Wiley & Sons Ltd.

LEARNING OUTCOMES

By the end of this chapter, you will have an understanding of the principles of continuous intravenous (IV) infusion.

A fluid or medicine administered over 24 hours via the IV route is referred to as a continuous IV infusion. These may be large volumes of fluid, such as 250–1000 ml, or small volumes, such as 50 ml. They may be repeated over days but delivered continuously.

Medications administered via continuous IV infusion may be abbreviated in many reference books as **C IV infusion**. It is best practise to deliver continuous IV infusions through a pump, for safety.

ADVANTAGES OF CONTINUOUS INTRAVENOUS INFUSION

- It may be used to maintain stable therapeutic concentrations of medicines, such as antibiotics.
- The infusion rate can be titrated according to the patient's needs, such as insulin to maintain set blood glucose levels.
- It allows medications with a short elimination half-life to be administered, such as adrenaline infusions in cardiac patients.
- Medications may be less irritating to the patient than bolus administrations

DISADVANTAGES OF CONTINUOUS INTRAVENOUS INFUSION

- The infusion may be complicated to prepare, such as having to add antibiotics to bags of fluid.
- Practitioners need to be familiar with infusion equipment, such as syringe drivers and volumatic pumps.

- It may be time-consuming to monitor patients on continuous IV infusions.
- There is a higher risk of microbial and particulate contamination than in bolus administration.
- Microbial contamination may be extrinsic or intrinsic. Extrinsic means that the infection is introduced during use, whereas intrinsic mean that the infection was present in the apparatus or medicine before use.
- There is a higher risk of infection than with bolus administration due to solutions taking longer to 'run through' and the potential for microbes to grow.
- Large volumes of fluid may cause fluid overload in some patients.

CALCULATING THE RATE

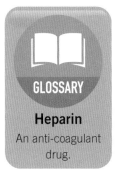

GLOSSARY

Heparin
An anti-coagulant drug.

Some drugs, such as heparin or an analgesic, need to be administered via specialised machinery, such as a syringe pump (Figure 12.1). These devices deliver set amounts of fluids, usually anything from 0.1 to 99 ml/h, of very concentrated drugs and with low flow rates. It is important that anyone using these devices undergoes specialist training, as there are many different devices used in clinical areas.

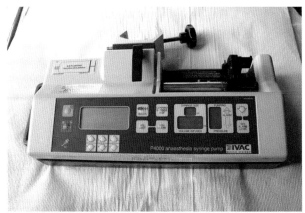

Figure 12.1 A syringe pump.

The formula for working out the IV infusion rate in millilitres per hour (with a syringe pump) is shown here:

$$\text{Infusion rate} = \frac{\text{amount of fluid (mL)}}{\text{Infusion time (hours)}}$$
$$= \text{millilitres per hour (pump)}$$

This can be shortened to:

$$\text{Rate} = \frac{\text{Volume}}{\text{Time}}$$

So, if I had 48 ml of fluid in my syringe to be delivered over 24 hours, I would input:

$$\frac{48\ \text{mL}}{24\ \text{hours}} = 2\ \text{mL/hour}$$

Therefore I would set the machine to deliver 2 ml/h, and after 24 hours my syringe would be empty.

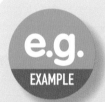

Let me show you an example. . . with insulin

Figures 12.2 and 12.3 are examples of the documentation that is used for patients with Type 1 diabetes. As you can see, we can record our patients' blood glucose levels. Insulin is administered subcutaneously.

If our patient then needs to receive their insulin via a continuous pump, they will be prescribed a set insulin regime and documentation with 'pump observations'. This way, their insulin can be titrated according to the blood glucose reading. This is known as a **sliding scale**. We can raise or lower the insulin dose the patient receives according to their blood glucose reading and the prescribed protocol. This mode of administration is by the IV route and is a temporary measure.

To prepare this infusion, I would need to wash my hands, put on an apron and gloves and clean my injection tray. I would need to gather all my equipment, insulin, syringe, needles and normal saline (or NS) and place these on the injection tray. I would need to check that my patient has a patent cannula and check for any signs of phlebitis. I would then recheck the prescription chart and ask a colleague to assist.

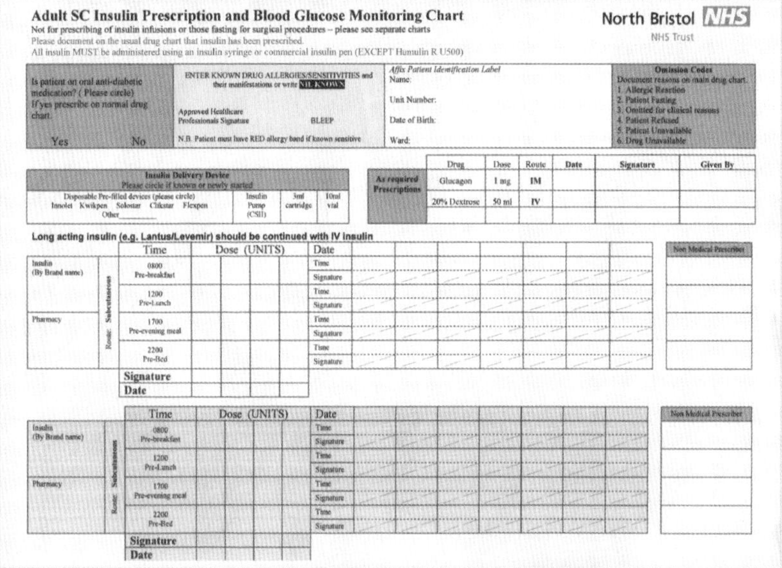

Adult SC Insulin Prescription and Blood Glucose Monitoring Chart

North Bristol NHS
NHS Trust

Not for prescribing of insulin infusions or those fasting for surgical procedures – please see separate charts
Please document on the usual drug chart that insulin has been prescribed.
All insulin MUST be administered using an insulin syringe or commercial insulin pen (EXCEPT Humulin R U500)

Is patient on oral anti-diabetic medication? (Please circle) If yes prescribe on normal drug chart. Yes No

ENTER KNOWN DRUG ALLERGIES/SENSITIVITIES and their manifestations or write NIL KNOWN
Approved Healthcare Professionals Signature BLEEP
N.B. Patient must have RED allergy band if known sensitive

Affix Patient Identification Label
Name:
Unit Number:
Date of Birth:
Ward:

Omission Codes
Document reasons on main drug chart.
1. Allergic Reaction
2. Patient Fasting
3. Omitted for clinical reasons
4. Patient Refused
5. Patient Unavailable
6. Drug Unavailable

Insulin Delivery Device
Please circle if known or newly started
Disposable Pre-filled devices (please circle) Innolet Kwikpen Solostar Clikstar Flexpen Other____ | Insulin Pump (CSII) | 3ml cartridge | 10ml vial

As required Prescriptions	Drug	Dose	Route	Date	Signature	Given By
	Glucagon	1 mg	IM			
	20% Dextrose	50 ml	IV			

Long acting insulin (e.g. Lantus/Levemir) should be continued with IV insulin

Insulin (By Brand name) / Pharmacy / Route: Subcutaneous
Time: 0800 Pre-breakfast; 1200 Pre-Lunch; 1700 Pre-evening meal; 2200 Pre-Bed
Dose (UNITS) / Date / Time / Signature / Non Medical Prescriber
Signature / Date

Insulin (By Brand name) / Pharmacy / Route: Subcutaneous
Time: 0800 Pre-breakfast; 1200 Pre-Lunch; 1700 Pre-evening meal; 2200 Pre-Bed
Dose (UNITS) / Date / Time / Signature / Non Medical Prescriber
Signature / Date

Figure 12.2 Adult SC insulin prescription and blood glucose monitoring chart. Source: Permission to reproduce this image is granted by North Bristol NHS Trust and University Hospitals Bristol NHS Foundation Trust.

The prescription is for Actrapid. The vials we have in stock are 1000 units/10 ml. I check this is an acceptable dose and, when I am satisfied, I draw up 50 units of the insulin into an insulin syringe.

I then draw up the normal saline into a 50 ml syringe. I inject the insulin into the normal saline syringe. This 50 ml syringe will now need to be gently inverted to mix the contents well.

Did you remember to make room for the insulin in the 50 ml syringe? This is the total amount we require in our syringe. The final volume of the syringe should be 50 ml and not a drop over (or under).

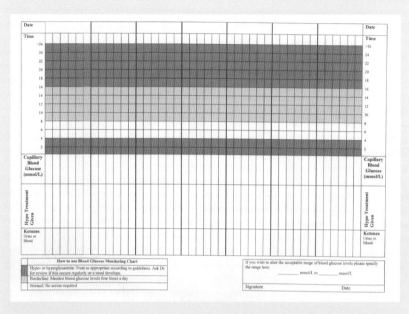

Figure 12.3 Blood glucose monitoring chart continuous IV infusion of insulin. Source: Permission to reproduce this image is granted by North Bristol NHS Trust and University Hospitals Bristol NHS Foundation Trust.

Our syringe contains 1 unit insulin to every 1 ml of fluid.

If we have started this continuous infusion because our patient is going into surgery, we usually set the infusion rate for our diabetic patients at:

Adults   2–4 units/h
Children   0.05 units/kg/h

But you will need to check the prescription and local protocol for this.

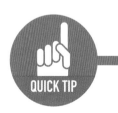

QUICK TIP

You may still see some medics writing units on prescription charts as IU, meaning International Units. This can be confused with IV for intravenous, so the word units is now preferred.

Don't confuse units with millilitres!

DIABETIC EMERGENCIES

First you will need to check local policies and procedures, but the usual initial infusion rates in adults in diabetic emergencies, known as diabetic ketoacidosis, is 6 units by IV bolus followed by 6 units/h by continuous infusion.

TEST YOUR KNOWLEDGE

1   Heparin is dispensed as 25 000 units in 1 ml. 20 000 IU of heparin is prescribed, to be diluted to 48 ml and administered over 24 h.
    (a)   What volume of heparin is required?
    (b)   How much dilutant is required?
    (c)   At what rate should the infusion pump be set?
2   An insulin infusion containing 50 units of human Actrapid has been diluted with 50 ml of sodium chloride, which has been running at:
    3 m/h for 3 hours
    3.5 m/h for 2 hours
    2 m/h for 2 hours
    2.5 ml/hour for 1 hour
    4 ml/hour for 1 hour

    How many units of Actrapid insulin in total has the patient received?

KEY POINTS

- The principles of administering drugs via continuous IV infusion.
- How to calculate drug rates in millilitres per hour.
- The principles of insulin sliding scales.

WEB RESOURCES

BNF: www.bnf.nice.org.uk
Pharmacy: www.rpharms.com

Chapter 13
· ·
ADMINISTRATION VIA PERCUTANEOUS ENDOSCOPIC GASTROSTOMY, PERCUTANEOUS ENDOSCOPIC JEJUNOSTOMY, OR NASOGASTRIC TUBE

Medicine Management Skills for Nurses, Second Edition. Claire Boyd.
© 2022 John Wiley & Sons Ltd. Published 2022 by John Wiley & Sons Ltd.

LEARNING OUTCOMES

By the end of this chapter, you will have an understanding of the administation of medications via percutaneous endoscopic gastrostomy (PEG), percutaneous endoscopic jejunostomy (PEJ), or nasogastric tube.

Individuals who are unable to swallow or maintain an adequate nutritional status, medication, and nutritional support may be fed or given their medications via:

- PEG tube,
- PEJ tube,
- nasogastric tube.

Collectively, these are known as **enteral feeding tubes** (Table 13.1).

GLOSSARY

Enteral
Relating to the intestinal tract.

Table 13.1 Enteral feeding tubes.

Enteral feeding tube	What you'll see on the prescription chart	What is it?
Percutaneous endoscopic gastrostomy tube	PEG	Patients who require longer-term enteral feeding (more than 4 wk) will require a PEG. A balloon holds the tube in position. The tube goes through the skin into the stomach.
Percutaneous endoscopic jejunostomy tube	PEJ	The tube goes through the skin into the loop of the jejunum. It is useful for patients who have severe delayed gastric emptying. Usually, the tube has a fine bore.

Enteral feeding tube	What you'll see on the prescription chart	What is it?
Nasogastric tube	NG	Suitable for short-term enteral feeding (less than four weeks). A wire introducer is supplied with many of these tubes to aid the intubation. The tube goes into the nose and down into the stomach. The position of the tube is checked by aspirating the gastric contents to establish a pH of less than 4, and auscultation of the epigastrium or X-ray. The end of the tube sits in the stomach.

MEDICATION

When administering drugs down these tubes, it should be remembered that most drugs are not licensed for administration via these routes. Common practice has been to crush medication designed for oral usage, which may result in tube blockage.

Also, for drugs that need to be given on an empty stomach feeding will need to be stopped for an appropriate time.

The tube should be flushed before and after the medication has been administered with at least 10 ml of water to clear the tube, but preferably 30 ml.

For patients requiring more than one drug at a time, the medications will need to be given separately and flushed between each administration with at least 10 ml of water.

All these amounts of water should be recorded on a fluid chart, including any enteral feeding regime that has been prescribed. Patients whose fluids have been restricted will be on a prescribed regime.

ADVICE FROM THE NPSA

The UK National Patient Safety Agency (NPSA) has advised health carers that:

Nasogastric tubes are not flushed, nor any liquid/feed introduced through the tube following initial placement, until the tube tip is confirmed by pH testing or X-ray to be in the stomach (Patient Safety Alert NPSA/2011/PSA002, NPSA, www.nrls.npsa.nhs.uk/resources/type/alerts/?entryid45=129640).

In addition:

The NPSA is aware of two patient deaths since 10 March 2011 where staff had flushed nasogastric tubes with water before initial placement had been confirmed. Staff then aspirated back the water they had flushed into the tube, including the lubricant within the tube that this water had activated. Because this mix of water and lubricant gave a pH reading below 5.5, they assumed that the nasogastric tube was correctly placed and went on to give medications and/or feed, although the tube was actually in the patient's lung. We are also aware of a similar incident which did not lead to harm to a patient (Harm from Flushing of Nasogastric Tubes before Confirmation of Placement, NPSA, www.nrls.npsa.nhs.uk/resources/?EntryId45=133441).

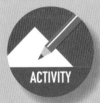

Activity 13.1

Why is it so important to establish placement of tube before administering feeds or medication down the tubes?

PLACEMENT OF TUBES

Figures 13.1 and 13.2 show the routes of short-and long-term nutrition support.

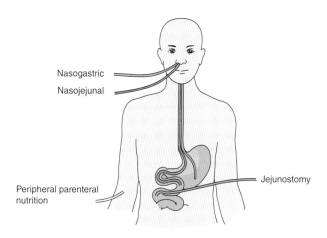

Figure 13.1 Routes of short-term nutritional support. NBT Enteral Feeding Policy (2009). Source: Permission to reproduce this image is granted by North Bristol NHS Trust and University Hospitals Bristol NHS Foundation Trust.

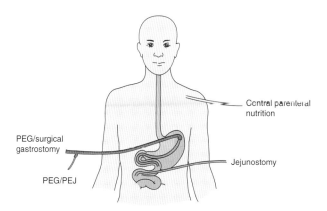

Figure 13.2 Routes of long-term nutritional support. NBT Enteral Feeding Policy (2009). Source: Permission to reproduce this image is granted by North Bristol NHS Trust and University Hospitals Bristol NHS Foundation Trust.

PARENTERAL NUTRITION

Parenteral nutrition (PN) is when nourishment is administered into a vein. Some patients are still able to eat and drink, but not enough to sustain life. Others who are unable to eat and drink receive all their nutrition this way and this is called **total parental nutrition** (or TPN). Some patients have their nutrition administered via a central venous catheter (CVC) directly into a large central vein.

Some of the names of the lines that you may hear are the PICC line (for peripherally inserted central catheter) or a Hickman line. The type of line – known as a CVC – may depend on whether PN is required by the patient in the long or the short term. Only after training can registered nurses deliver drugs or nutrition down a CVC device, but students can of course observe the procedure if the patient consents to you doing so. TPN requires close monitoring.

ENTERAL FEEDING REGIMES

The dietician will prescribe a feeding regime to suit the patient. A selection of these can be seen in Table 13.2.

Table 13.2 An example of an enteral feeding regime.

Feed	Type	Kcal/ml
Nutrison	Whole protein	1.0
Nutrison multifibre	Whole protein, fibre	1.0
Nutrison energy	Whole protein	1.5
Nutrison energy multifibre	Whole protein fibre	1.5
Nutrison protein plus	Whole protein, high protein	1.25
Nutrison advanced cubison	Whole protein, very high protein	1.0
Nutrison concentrated	Whole protein, low fluid	2.0
Nutrison peptisorb	Predigested protein	1.0

Methods of Administering Enteral Feeds

There are many enteral feeding pumps on the market, with a range of flow rates from 1 to 300 ml per hour. Some feeds may be decanted into PVC (polyvinyl chloride) bags or bottles.

Feeding regimes can be administered by:

- Continuous feeding via a pump,
- Intermittent feeding via gravity,
- Intermittent feeding via a pump,
- Bolus feeding.

Procedure for Nasogastric Intubation

The procedure and equipment for nasogastric intubation are outlined in Table 13.3.

Table 13.3 Procedure and equipment for nasogastric intubation.

Equipment required
1 nasogastric tube
50 ml oral/enteral syringe (purple)
Glass of orange juice/squash and straw (*only* if you cannot obtain a pH less than or equal to 4 and the patient has a 'safe' swallow)
Penlight
Tissues
pH strip (3 pad, pH 2–9)
Disposable gloves (sterile if immunocompromised) and apron
Water (sterile if immunocompromised)
Vomit bowl

Intervention	Rationale
1 Check with patient and hospital notes for any contraindications.	To minimise risk of potential problems.
2 Explain the procedure and obtain verbal consent. Arrange a signal the patient can use to slow or stop proceedings.	To reduce anxiety and gain consent.
3 Position patient in a semi-upright position if able (not spinal patients), with the head tilted slightly forward to reduce cervical flexure (Figure 13.3).	This will reduce the risk of tracheal intubation but increases the chance of oesophageal intubation.

(*Continued*)

Table **13.3** (*Continued*)

Intervention	Rationale
Check the following: determine the length of tube for insertion. This is done by measuring from the xiphisternum to the ear, then to the ear to the nose, plus 5 cm. This measurement is known as the *limiting mark* (Figure 13.4).	
4 Wash hands with soap and water and put on apron and gloves.	To minimize the risk of cross-infection.
5 Inject 10 ml of tap water and dip in the tip of the tube.	For ease of insertion and patient comfort during procedure.
6 Check the nostrils for polyps or deviated septum by asking the patient to alternately blow out of each nostril, if able.	For patient comfort.
7 Gently insert 10 cm of the tube, directing horizontally. Ask patient to gently start humming.	This opens the nasopharynx by lowering the soft palate.
8 Continue passing, without hesitation, until reaching the limiting mark. Secure tube.	For correct positioning of tube and patient safety.
9 Make the patient comfortable.	For patient comfort.
10 Remove gloves and apron (place in a clinical waste bag) and wash your hands.	To prevent cross-contamination.
11 Record the administration of the medication on the prescription chart.	To keep accurate documentation.

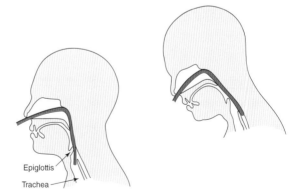

Epiglottis

Trachea

Figure 13.3 Head position during nasogastric intubation. NBT Enteral Feeding Policy (2009). Source: Permission to reproduce this image is granted by North Bristol NHS Trust and University Hospitals Bristol NHS Foundation Trust.

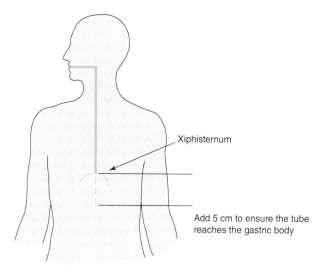

Xiphisternum

Add 5 cm to ensure the tube
reaches the gastric body

Figure 13.4 Finding the limiting mark; measure from
xiphisternum to ear to nose. NBT Enteral Feeding Policy
(2009). Source: Permission to reproduce this image is
granted by North Bristol NHS Trust and University Hospitals
Bristol NHS Foundation Trust.

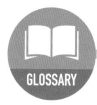

GLOSSARY

Xiphisternum
The lowermost section of the breastbone.

Procedure for Securing the Tube

The guidewire should be withdrawn during intubation only
when the nasogastric position has been confirmed.

The tube should be taped to the nose and cheek using a
tape-bridge (Figure 13.5). The tube should not be taped on
the forehead as this may obstruct the patient's vision. Using
a tape bridge will reduce the risk of nasal erosion.

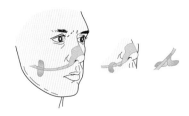

Figure 13.5 Securing the tube. NBT Enteral Feeding Policy (2009). Source: Permission to reproduce this image is granted by North Bristol NHS Trust and University Hospitals Bristol NHS Foundation Trust.

Mark the tube at the nose, known as the limiting mark (Figure 13.4), so that any slippage can be spotted and acted on.

NASOGASTRIC CARE PLAN

Patients with an enteral feeding tube will require careful documentation of the care of this tube. Figure 13.6 shows a typical example of a Nasogastric Tube Care Plan.

TEST YOUR KNOWLEDGE

A patient has had a nasogastric tube inserted. You collect the prescription chart and see that the patient has been prescribed the following drugs. Can they be crushed and put down the tube?

Propranolol capsules, modified release (for hypertension)

Zopiclone tablets, whole tablet (for insomnia)

Lactulose solution (for constipation)

Fluoxetine capsule (for depression)

Actrapid insulin, 4 units SC (for Type 1 diabetes)

Reason for Nasogastric Tube..........................

Affix patient label

Type of tube.....................Date inserted...................

PH on insertion...................Limiting mark...................cm

Referral to Dietician

Sign..................... Date...................

Referral to Speech and Language therapist if appropriate

Sign..................... Date...................

	Date	E	L	N	E	L	N	E	L	N	E	L	N	E	L	N
	Action															
1	*Hand hygiene*															
	Wash hands and wear non-sterile gloves prior to manipulating tube															
2	*Patient hygiene and comfort*															
	Inspect mouth & provide regular mouth-care															
	Clean nostrils daily and change adhesive tape if soiled															
	Ensure tube is well secured in place on face/cheek/nose															
	Rotate external position of the tube and check for pressure damage															

Figure 13.6 (*Continued*)

	Action	E	L	N	E	L	N	E	L	N	E	L	N	E	L	N
3	**Tube position** Check limiting mark on tube is in correct position and record this in cm here every shift. Refer to policy if evidence of malposition. Check position of NG tube prior to administration of feed, drugs, at least once during each continuous feeding episode and after violent coughing or obvious tube movement. Check gastric aspirate 4 hourly to confirm stomach position, and indicate which confirmation method below is used:															
	a. pH less than or equal to 4															
	b. pH less than or equal to 4 after patient drank half-diluted orange squash															
	c. pH less than 5 & aspirate is 'grass green' or more than 10ml															
	d. pH less than 5 & patient on ranitidine/omeprazole/lansoprazole															
	e. No confirmation but tube position unchanged: i.e. limiting mark still at nose, no coil in nasopharynx, no evidence of regurgitation															
	f. If steps above fail a Trained operator must use a Cortrak trace if available or X-ray to confirm gastric position and record in patient record and sign here................Time................															
4	**Enteral Feeding** If receiving feed via a pump ensure the patient is positioned at 30 degree angle															

Figure 13.6 (*Continued*)

Action	E	L	N	E	L	N	E	L	N	E	L	N	E	L	N
Ensure enteral feeding syringes are used and changed every 24 hours															
Feed giving sets must be changed every 24 hours and unused feed discarded															
If having bolus feeds partially used bottles to be returned to the fridge & discarded after 24 hours															
Do not re-use single use items such as syringes and reservoirs/ hydrobags															
5 Fluid and nutrition recording															
Maintain fluid balance chart, record all feed related input and output including hourly feed rate & total volume delivered															
Complete food chart if patient is eating, include supplements															
Follow prescribed dietetic feeding regime or emergency feeding protocol if out of hours/weekend															
Document weekly weight on the malnutrition screening tool															
6 Medication via nasogastric tubes															
Only administer soluble medication or finely crushed tablets at the instruction of a pharmacist															
Mix medication with 10–15 mL of water and give each drug separately															
Flush tube before and after medication with at least 10 mL of water															

Figure 13.6 Nasogastric tube care plan (for all types of nasogastric tube). NBT Enteral Feeding Policy (2009). Source: Permission to reproduce this Image is granted by North Bristol NHS Trust and University Hospitals Bristol NHS Foundation Trust.

KEY POINTS

- Types of enteral feeding tubes and their placement.
- The administration of medications down enteral tubes.
- Principles of parenteral and TPN.
- Principles of nasogastric intubation and securing the tube.
- Nasogastric tube documentation.

WEB RESOURCES

BNF Adults: www.bnf.nice.org.uk
BNF Children: www.bnfc.nice.org.uk
The Royal Marsden Clinical Nursing Procedures:
 www.rmmonline.co.uk/manual
You will need to register and log in.
National Patient Safety Agency: www.npsa.nhs.uk

RESOURCES

NBT Enteral Feeding Policy 2009,North Bristol NHS Trust
and University Hospitals Bristol NHS Foundation, Bristol

Chapter 14
OXYGEN THERAPY

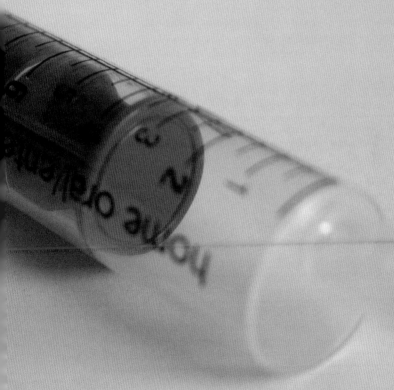

Medicine Management Skills for Nurses, Second Edition. Claire Boyd.
© 2022 John Wiley & Sons Ltd. Published 2022 by John Wiley & Sons Ltd.

LEARNING OUTCOMES

By the end of this chapter you will have an understanding of factors relating to oxygen therapy, such as respiration, proning, symptoms of hypoxaemia, and hypercapnoea, oxygen administration devices, titrating oxygen therapy, and monitoring.

Not all medicines come out of bottles or blister packages. Oxygen Therapy, also known as supplemental oxygen, is the use of oxygen as a medical treatment. Oxygen therapy is believed to be the most common treatment administered in hospital and is listed on the World Health Organisations (WHO) 21st list of **essential medicines.** It is widely used in hospital and home settings and is classified as a medical gas. Just like any drug, it should always be remembered that excessively high amounts, or concentrations, can cause harm due to oxygen toxicity. The National Patient Safety Agency (overseers of healthcare) have identified problems in four areas of oxygen therapy:

- Prescription
- Administration
- Monitoring
- Equipment.

There are tools to assist the safe administration of oxygen therapy:

- Prescription charts
- Oxygen monitors (pulse oximetry)
- News II observation chart
- Oxygen mask/device.
- Training for those who administer oxygen.

Before looking at the aims of oxygen therapy and the administration, it is first important we have a quick overview of the physiology of breathing.

RESPIRATION

Lets start with the basics: Normal breathing acts to do two things:

- Get oxygen into the body – which is necessary for the respiration of cells.
- Get carbon dioxide out of the body – which is produced as a waste product.

The more work the cells are doing, the more oxygen they will require and the more carbon dioxide they will produce, thus the more carbon dioxide they will produce, thus the more breathing is necessary.

Oxygen is required for normal cell metabolism. A lack of oxygen means:

- Cells can't function normally.
- Can lead to cell damage and death.
- Can lead to organ damage and death.
- Can lead to patient damage and death.

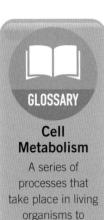

GLOSSARY

Cell Metabolism

A series of processes that take place in living organisms to sustain those organisms.

What Happens When We Breath?

Breathing in (inspiration)	The diaphragm flattens and the ribs elevate, Which increases the volume of the thoracic cavity; air moves into the lungs.
Breathing out (expiration)	The diaphragm and the ribs return to their normal positions decreasing the volume of the thoracic cavity; air moves out of the lungs.

The aim of inspiration is to move air to the area of the lung where gas exchange can take place. This is in the air sacs (alveoli). Gas exchange can be aided by patient positioning, such as sitting the patient up, using pillows, angling the bed and proning.

What Is Proning?

Proning is the process of turning a patient with precise, safe motions from their back onto their abdomen (stomach) so that the individual is lying face down.

It is effective at boosting 'blood oxygen saturation' levels among covid patients struggling with abnormally low levels (known as hypoxia).

Proning is used in patients with severe Acute Respiratory Distress Syndrome (ARDS) and hypoxemia, which is not improved by other means. It is beneficial for the patient due to;

- Better ventilation of the dorsal lung regions threatened by alveolar collapse.
- Improvement in ventilation/perfusion.
- Potentially an improvement in mortality.

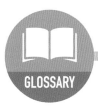

GLOSSARY

ARDS = Respiratory failure characterised by rapid onset of widespread inflammation in the lungs. Symptoms include shortness of breath, rapid breathing, bluish skin colouration.

Dorsal = Situated at the back.

Alveolar = Relating to the alveoli of the lung/s. Alveoli (plural) are the tiny air sacs of the lungs which allow for rapid gaseous exchange.

Mortally = Death.

What Makes Us Breath?

Breathing is under the control of the nervous system. The most important trigger for breathing is raised carbon dioxide levels in the blood. If we produce more carbon dioxide (e.g. through exercise) this is sensed and causes an increased respiratory rate. We also have receptors which sense low oxygen levels. If oxygen levels decrease this will also stimulate breathing – this is less important mechanism in healthy people.

Some patients (particularly those with long term conditions affecting the lungs or breathing muscles) become accustomed to high carbon dioxide levels. This then stops acting as a trigger to breathe.

These patients also become accustomed to lower oxygen levels. Low oxygen levels become the trigger to breathe in these patients.

If these patients are given too much oxygen, the oxygen levels in their blood rises. This can cause these people to lose their respiratory drive. Their respiratory rate gradually falls, carbon dioxide levels rise and the patient can lose consciousness and die.

Who Is at Risk of Respiratory Failure

- Chronic Obstructive Pulmonary Disease (COPD)
- Cystic Fibrosis (CF)
- Non-CF Bronchiectasis
- Kyphoscoliosis/ankylosing spondylitis
- Severe scarring from TB (tuberculosis)
- Morbid obesity
- Musculoskeletal disorders

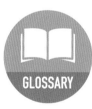

GLOSSARY

Kyphoscoliosis
A disorder of the spine, involving abnormal curvature.

Ankylosing Spondylitis
A type of arthritis in the spine causing inflammation and gradual fusing of the vertebrae.

One of the facts about Covid 19 patients is that they often presented in hospitals unaware that their oxygen levels were so dangerously low.

What Are the Physical Symptoms of Low Oxygen (Hypoxaemia) or High Carbon Dioxide (Hypercapnoea)?

Hypoxaemia

- Breathlessness
- Agitation
- Confusion
- Tachycardia

- Tachypnoea
- Physical tiredness
- Increased work of breathing
- Increased or decreased ventilation

Hypercapnoea

- Drowsiness (Decrease ACVPU)
- Headaches
- Respiratory distress
- Flushed face
- Warm peripheries
- Full and bounding pulse
- Confusion
- Muscle twitching
- Outstretched hands
- Convulsions
- Coma

Certain medical conditions lead to decreased function of the lungs and low oxygen levels:

- Pneumonia
- Pulmonary oedema
- Pulmonary fibrosis
- Pneumothorax
- Pulmonary embolism
- ARDS
- Crushed chest injury
- Poisoning
- Exacerbations of underlying lung disease
- Covid 19

Supplementally oxygen is required for these patients to maintain their oxygen saturation levels. This is delivered via wall oxygen delivery systems or free standing gas cylinders. The amount of oxygen used is guided by the individuals saturations levels, and the pressure flow is controlled by a flowmeter in most cases and is measured in litres per minute (lpm). The effectiveness of the supplemental oxygen is measured by recording saturations. Depending on whether the patient is at risk of respiratory failure or not affects the target saturations.

ADMINISTERING THE OXYGEN

Below is a visual representation of delivering oxygen to patients. Figure 14.1

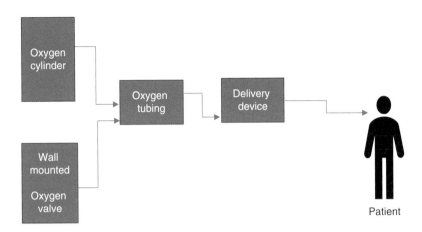

Figure 14.1 Oxygen administration.

To deliver oxygen effectively to patients, or the home user, the correct delivery device should be used. There are many types of delivery device, delivering varying amounts of oxygen, such as:

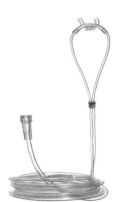

- Nasal cannula (also known as nasal specs or spigs)
- Simple masks (such as a Hudson mask)
- Non-rebreathe Masks (with reservoir bag)
- Venturi devices (used to deliver specific amounts of oxygen)

Nasal Cannula

This device is a thin tube with two small nozzles or spigs that protrude into the persons nostrils. They provide oxygen at low flow rates at 1–6lpm, delivering concentrations of 24–44%. They are more comfortable than other devices and less intrusive than masks. Figure 14.2 shows a Nasal Cannula.

Figure 14.2 Nasal cannula.

The downfall of these devices is that:

- The inspired oxygen rate varies widely depending on the person's respiratory rate
- Some patients are mouth breathers
- The drying effect to the mucous membranes
- Can't use these devices with a blocked nose

Simple Masks

There are many varieties of masks used in practice, often delivering 5–8lpm, with concentrations of anything between 28% and 50%

Non - rebreathe Masks

These masks use a reservoir bag to pool the oxygen. Figure 14.3 shows a non - rebreathe masks.

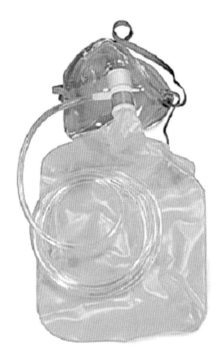

Figure 14.3 Non - rebreathe masks.

These devices deliver >90% oxygen therapy and are used with 15 lpm. They are designed to draw oxygen from the attached reservoir bag, with one-way valves that direct exhaled air out of the mask, preventing exhaled air from returning to the bag. The reservoir bag must be filled prior to use. This type of mask is indicated for acute medical emergencies but can be claustrophobic for the patient and the delivery varies with the mask fit.

High flow oxygen therapy is generally used for the following situations:

- Cardiac-Arrest/Resuscitation
- Major trauma
- Near-drowning
- Major head injury
- Carbon-Monoxide poisoning
- Covid 19 patients

All other situations, the aim is to maintain target situations, which are generally:

94–98% in most patients
92–98% in those over 70 years of age
88–92% in those with risk factors for respiratory failure.

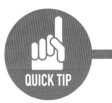

QUICK TIP

REMEMBER: Levels of oxygen that are too high can be as bad as levels that are too low. For accurate assessment of oxygen recordings, blood samples are taken – known as ABGs (arterial blood gas)

Venturi Mask Valves

These are controlled air-entrainment masks, known as venturi masks, which can accurately deliver a predetermined oxygen concentration of up to 60%. They work by mixing the oxygen with room air in the valve and they are colour coded with the oxygen flow rate written on the side of the valve. Figure 14.4 shows the working mechanism of the venturi valve.

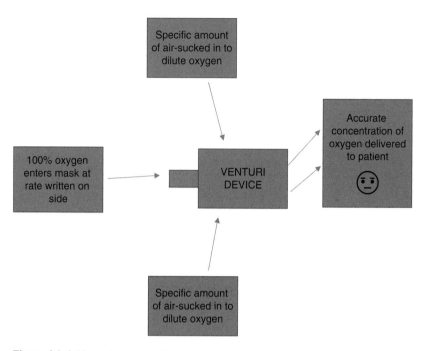

Figure 14.4 Venturi valve working mechanism.

Venturi mask valves have standard colour coding with four of the most common devices:

Blue = 24%

Yellow = 35%
Red = 40%

There is also an orange valve which delivers 31% and a green valve which delivers 60% oxygen.

Titrating Oxygen Therapy

This is about maintaining the patients target oxygen saturations – administering more oxygen therapy or less oxygen therapy as their condition detects. Figure 14.5 shows how to titrate oxygen therapy.

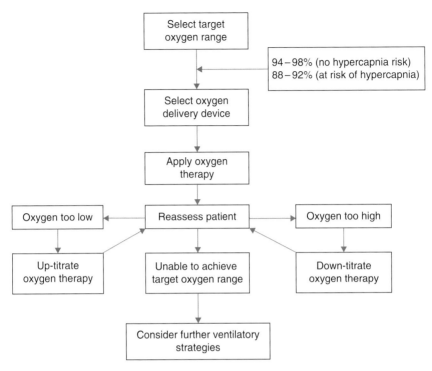

Figure 14.5 Oxygen titration.

DETERIORATING PATIENTS

One aspect of treating a patient with oxygen deterioration may follow these oxygen therapy steps:

Nasal cannulae 1 lpm
Nasal cannulae 2 lpm
Nasal cannulae 4 lpm
24% Venturi (blue)
28% Venturi (white)
35% Venturi (yellow)
40% Venturi (red)
Non re-breathe Reservoir Mask 15 lpm

SIGNS OF RESPIRATORY DETERIORATION

These symptoms should raise suspicion of worsening respiratory function, as monitoring those we care for is not all about machine monitoring but using our observation and communication skills:

- Oxygen decreased by >3%
- Increasing oxygen requirements
- Increasing News II score
- Carbon Dioxide retention with pH < 7.35
- Drowsiness
- Headache
- Tremor

Appropriate action would include changing the oxygen delivery but first alerting medical staff.

OXYGEN CYLINDERS

Cylinders, as opposed to piped wall oxygen, are a limited source of oxygen, useful for home use or transferring patients in a hospital setting. They will become empty faster when being used by patients using higher flow rates, and of course with cylinders of smaller capacities. It should also be remembered that when picking up any cylinder, they need to be checked first as they may not be full to start with, and that different manufacturers may use different cylinder capacities. Below shows cylinder capacity flow rates Figure 14.6

Within hospitals and care settings, oxygen and medical air delivery systems are wall mounted and these ports can look similar. It can therefore be easy to mistake one for the other. Figure 14.7 shows the wall ports, with flow meters attached.

Hospital Patients

Every patient should have their target saturations prescribed by medical staff on admission.

Cylinder size	CD	E	HX	G	J
Gas type	Oxygen	Oxygen	Oxygen	Oxygen	Oxygen
Capacity(l)	460.0	680.0	2300	3400	6800
Flow Rate(l)	(h)	(h)	(h)	(h)	(h)
1.00	7.7	11.3	38.3	56.7	113.3
2.00	3.8	5.7	19.2	28.3	56.7
3.00	2.6	3.8	12.8	18.9	37.8
4.00	1.9	2.8	9.6	14.2	28.3
5.00	1.5	2.3	7.7	11.3	22.7
6.00	1.3	1.9	6.4	9.4	18.9
7.00	1.1	1.6	5.5	8.1	16.2
8.00	1.0	1.4	4.8	7.1	14.2
9.00	0.9	1.3	4.3	6.3	12.6
10.00	0.8	1.1	3.8	5.7	11.3
11.00	0.7	1.0	3.5	5.2	10.3
12.00	0.6	0.9	3.2	4.7	9.4
13.00	0.6	0.9	2.9	4.4	8.7
14.00	0.5	0.8	2.7	4.0	8.1
15.00	0.5	0.8	2.6	3.8	7.6

Cylinder capacity (litres)/Flow rate (lpm)/60 = hours supply

Figure 14.6 Examples of oxygen cylinder capacity rates.

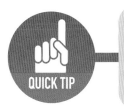

QUICK TIP

Oxygen Therapy is a prescribed drug.

Oxygen must not be administered without a prescription, except in resuscitation situations.

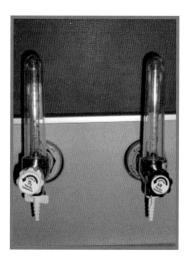

Figure 14.7 Wall ports, with flow meters attached.

The medical staff will take into account the patient's risk of respiratory failure. The prescribed oxygen is documented on the NEWS II observation chart as a scale 1 or scale 2. The NEWS II observation chart can be seen at www.rcplondon. ac.uk/projects/outputs/national-early-warning-score-news.

Scale 1

- Used for patients **NOT** at risk of hypercapnic respiratory failure
- Determined by Oxygen Prescription in drug chart being completed indicating Scale 1
- Record saturations with a **number**
- If oxygen **not** prescribed, Scale 1 will be the default until the doctor completes the drug chart oxygen section

Scale 2

- Used for patients **WITH** or **AT HIGH** risk of hypercapnic respiratory failure (often patients with COPD, neuro-muscular disease, morbid obesity).
- Only a Doctor, Site Nurse Practitioner, or Specialist Nurse from the respiratory team can authorise the use of scale 2.

- This decision must clearly documented and signed in the:
    - **Observation chart**
    - **Prescription chart**
    - **Patient Notes**
- Record saturations with a **number.**

APPROACH TO MONITORING

Oxygen Saturations should be measured in all breathless patients and all patients on oxygen. This monitoring is conducted using a pulse oximetry device. Oxygen saturations should be adjusted to keep the saturations within the target prescribed and measured continuously for five minutes after any change in oxygen adnistered.

CASE STUDY

Let me show you how all the information we have covered in this chapter can be put into practise with our patient Michael Rogers. Tyler Winters is a Nursing Associate and is reading what the Medic has just written in this patients notes:

Name: Micheal Rogers
Gender: Male
Age: 74-year-old
Past Medical History: COPD – on regular inhalers
Normal exercise tolerance 20/30 yards
Heavy smoker for 50 years+
Medications: Combivent Nebulisers
Seretide inhalers
Tiotropium inhalers
Prednisolone
Bendrofluazide
Augmentin
Clarithromycin
Allergies: None Known
No pain. Discomfort on breathing
Anxious/Restless
Pulling off Nasal specs

Observations:

RR: 40 bpm
SpO2: 82% Scale 2
Oxygen Therapy: 4l via nasal specs
Target saturations: 88–92%
BP: 145/80
HR: 130
ACVPU: Confused (New)
Temperature: 38 °C
NEWS SCORE: 13

The Medic is writing the prescription chart for the patient to be given medications to relieve their symptoms and at the same time organises a treatment plan for this patient. This is what we would expect Michael Rogers's care management to look like:

- Titrate oxygen therapy to venturi mask – 24%
- Raise patient to a sitting position
- Constant oxygen monitoring
- A – E assessment (NEWS II observation chart) Continuous monitoring
- Cannulate patient and take bloods
- Administer prescribed medications
- Cardiac Monitoring
- Reassure patient
- Record all information
- Target oxygen saturations for this patient are 88–92%

TEST YOUR KNOWLEDGE

1   What tools can be used to assist the safe administration of oxygen therapy?
2   What is 'proning'?
3   What are the physical symptoms of low oxygen levels in the body?
4   What is the percentage of oxygen able venturi mask valve can deliver?

KEY POINTS

- Looking at how to recognise respiratory failure hypoxaemia and hypercapnoea in patients
- Looking at how to administer oxygen devices and titrate oxygen therapy
- Looking at how to monitor oxygen saturation levels

WEB RESOURCES

NewsII:www.rcplondon.ac.uk/projects/outputs/national-early-warning-score-news

World Health Organisation: www.who.int

www.who.int/.../essential-medicines-list

National Patient Safety Agency: www.npsa.nhs.uk

Chapter 15
. . . .
DRUGS AND SPECIFIC
MEDICAL CONDITIONS

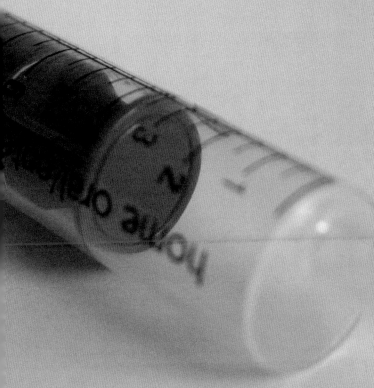

Medicine Management Skills for Nurses, Second Edition. Claire Boyd.
© 2022 John Wiley & Sons Ltd. Published 2022 by John Wiley & Sons Ltd.

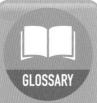

GLOSSARY

Prostaglandins

One of a group of hormone-like substances present in a wide variety of tissues and body fluids.

Depending on your clinical placement during your training, you will no doubt come across some very commonly prescribed drugs. It is recommended that you read more in depth about these drugs – their indications, cautions, contra-indications, side effects, and dosage – but here is a little taster.

ASPIRIN AND NSAIDs

Aspirin belongs to a group of analgesics known as the non-steroidal anti-inflammatory drugs, or NSAIDs. Specifically, it is in the salicylates category.

These drugs are used primarily to treat inflammation, mild to moderate pain and fever. During tissue injury prostaglandins are released, and NSAIDs can block the enzyme that synthesises prostaglandin, decreasing any associated inflammation and fever. Unfortunately, prostaglandins also have a protective role on the gastro-intestinal mucosa and the action of the NSAIDs contributes to the symptoms of dyspepsia, peptic erosions, and ulceration, hence the rationale for them often to be taken with food. Also, aspirin is contra-indicated in children under 12 years of age due to the possible risk of Reye's syndrome; this is characterised by brain and liver damage, but it is very rare.

Individuals who have a cardiovascular disease, such as angina, peripheral vascular disease, a previous heart attack, transient ischaemic attack (TIA) or cerebral vascular accident (CVA), may have been advised to take low-dose aspirin (75 mg) every day.

How Does Aspirin Work to Prevent Blood Clots?

Aspirin works to lower the risk of blood clots forming in the arteries in the heart or brain, which helps to prevent myocardial infarction (a heart attack) or cerebrovascular accident (stroke). Here's how clots are formed, and aspirin helps to prevent them:

1 A blood clot may form in an artery, preventing blood from adequately reaching the heart or brain.
2 Atheroma patches develop on the inside lining of some arteries, known as hardening of the arteries.
3 Platelets are particles in the blood that help the blood to clot when a blood vessel is cut: platelets sometimes stick to the atheroma inside the artery.
4 Low-dose aspirin reduces the stickiness of the platelets, which stops them from sticking to the atheroma in the vessel and forming a clot.

The side effects of aspirin include gastro-intestinal irritation, increased bleeding time, bronchospasms in people with asthma and skin reactions in hypersensitive individuals.

PARACETAMOL

Paracetamol (also known as acetaminophen) is an analgesic and an anti-pyretic (meaning that it lowers high temperature). It is a mainstay in many homes. Paracetamol comes in a variety of forms (tablets, capsules, dispersible, suspension, suppository, intravenous preparation), and brand names. Adults and children over three months old can take the drug up to four times a day, every four to six hours, for short periods of time. However, caution should be applied to those with hepatic impairment, renal impairment, and alcohol dependence. Paracetamol does not cause gastric irritation but is hepatotoxic in high doses. Many over-the-counter treatments for colds and influenza contain paracetamol, resulting in inadvertent overdoses that can cause death from liver failure. The antidote to paracetamol poisoning is acetylcysteine.

MONOAMINE OXIDASE INHIBITORS

Monoamine oxidase inhibitors, also known as MAOIs, are a group of drugs used in the treatment of depression that inhibit monoamine oxidase, an enzyme found in brain tissue. This causes an accumulation of amine neurotransmitters in the brain, relieving the depression. MAOIs may also be prescribed for patients with phobias, atypical hypochondria or features of hysteria.

The fact that MAOIs *inhibit* monoamine oxidase and cause amine neurotransmitters to accumulate gives rise to many safety concerns. As amine levels rise, if the patient eats one of the many foodstuffs containing the amine tyramine an anticholinergic reaction can occur, having a similar effect in the body to that of adrenaline. This can lead to hypertensive crisis, a dangerous rise in blood pressure. Foods containing tyramine include:

- Mature cheese,
- Pickled herring,
- Broad bean pods,
- Meat- and yeast-extract spreads.

Patients taking MAOIs are also advised to avoid stale food or foods that might be 'going off', and alcohol.

Prescribed MAOIs include:

- isocarboxazid,
- phenelzine,
- tranylcypromine.

These drugs tend to be increased slowly to the therapeutic dose, and due to the safety concerns MAOIs are usually prescribed when other antidepressants have not worked.

Side effects of MAOIs include daytime sleepiness, low blood pressure, dizziness, diarrhoea, dry mouth, muscle aches, altered sense of taste, nervousness, insomnia, weight gain, reduced sexual desire, erectile dysfunction, difficulty urinating, and paraesthesia to the skin.

THE CO-DRUGS

Many drugs contain two active ingredients. Table 15.1 lists some of these drugs.

Table **15.1** Some co-drugs.

Drug name	What is it?	Active ingredients
Co-amilofruse 2.5/20	Potassium-sparing diuretic with other diuretic	Amiloride hydrochloride 2.5 mg, furosemide 20 mg
Co-amilozide 2.5/25	Potassium-sparing diuretic with other diuretic	Amiloride hydrochloride 2.5 mg, hydrochlorothiazide 25 mg
Co-amoxiclav 250/125	Penicillin	Amoxicillin 250 mg, clavulanic acid 125 mg
Co-beneldopa 125	Dopaminergic drug used in Parkinsonism	Benserazide 25 mg, levodopa 100 mg
Co-careldopa 10/100	Dopaminergic drug used in Parkinsonism	Carbidopa 10 mg, levodopa 100 mg
Co-codamol 8/500	Analgesic	Codeine phosphate 8 mg, paracetamol 500 mg
Co-dydramol 10/500	Analgesic	Dihydrocodeine tartrate 10 mg, paracetamol 500 mg

As you can see, the drug name has a set of numbers after it. These relate to the doses of the active ingredients in the tablet or capsule.

The last two drugs – co-codamol and co-dydramol – contain paracetamol with an opioid analgesic. Opioid analgesics work by mimicking the action of our own naturally occurring pain chemicals, called endorphins, which are found in the brain and spinal cord. Endorphins combine with opioid receptors and reduce the pain.

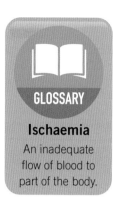

DRUGS USED IN SPECIFIC MEDICAL CONDITIONS

Cerebrovascular Accident: Stroke

There are two major types of stroke: ischaemic stroke and haemorrhagic stroke.

An ischaemic stroke (also known as a transient ischemic attack) occurs when blood flow to the brain is occluded by a blood clot. This may form two ways:

- Thrombotic stroke: formation of a clot in an already narrowed blood vessel.
- Embolic stroke: when a clot breaks off from another place in a blood vessel and travels to the brain.

A haemorrhagic stroke is caused when a blood vessel in the brain bursts, causing bleeding into the brain (known as an intracerebral haemorrhage) or around the brain, in the space between the brain and the skull (known as a subarachnoid haemorrhage). A subarachnoid haemorrhage can be caused by a bulge in the wall of an artery (an aneurysm) or a leakage from malformed blood vessels (known as an arteriovenous malformation, or AVM).

Symptoms of a haemorrhagic stroke vary depending on the type of stroke, and include (amongst others):

- intracerebral haemorrhage: sudden weakness, paralysis, or numbness in any part of the body, inability to speak and vomiting,
- subarachnoid haemorrhage (caused by a ruptured aneurysm): sudden severe headache, nausea, vomiting, stiff neck, dizziness, and seizure.

Table 15.2 lists the risk factors for having a stroke.

Treatment

A stroke is a medical emergency and immediate treatment can save lives and reduce disability. First the patient must

Table 15.2 Stroke risk factors.

High blood pressure	Diabetes
Atrial fibrillation	Family history of a stroke
High cholesterol	Increasing age (especially after 55 yr of age)
Ethnic origin: black people are more likely to experience a stroke	Being overweight or obese
Drinking heavily	Eating too much fat or salt
Smoking	Taking the birth control pill

undergo a CT scan to establish whether the stroke was caused by a clot or by bleeding. The patient must begin treatment within three hours of the stroke. If it was a ischaemic stroke then the patient should begin thrombolytic therapy, also known as 'clot-busting drugs'. The clot is broken down by these drugs and blood flow to the damaged area will re-commence. Other treatments may include heparin, warfarin, and aspirin.

If it was a haemorrhagic stroke instead of being caused by clotting, then thrombolytic drugs can cause more bleeding. Treatment for haemorrhagic strokes involves lowering the pressure in the skull. This pressure, known as the intracranial pressure (ICP), will need to be measured. A mechanical ventilator may be required to hyperventilate the patient. A drug known as mannitol may be prescribed which transports brain fluid into the bloodstream, again to lower the ICP. A surgeon may have to cut the skull bone to decrease the pressure in the brain, so that the swelling does not 'push down' into the brain stem (known as 'coning', and which is fatal). Some medics also prescribe anti-epileptic medication in case of seizures as a protective measure.

If the bleeding is caused by an AVM, surgery may be required to repair the abnormality. For aneurysms, an operation known as a 'clipping' or 'coiling' may be undertaken by a neurosurgeon to correct the problem. Following the procedures an intense course of occupational therapy and physiotherapy may be required due to any disability experienced during the brain assault.

Myocardial Infarction

Individuals who have experienced a myocardial infarction (or MI) will be advised to take certain medications for the rest of their lives to reduce the chance of another MI and to prevent their heart disease from getting worse. These drugs are:

- aspirin: to prevent blood clots,
- beta-blockers: to help to protect the heart,
- Angiotensin converting enzyme (ACE) inhibitors: to help protect the heart,
- statins: to lower cholesterol levels.

Beta-blockers ease the workload of the heart by blocking the beta receptors on the muscle cells of heart. When the beta receptors are stimulated – by the hormones adrenaline and noradrenaline – they make the heart work harder, which increases heart rate and blood pressure. Beta-blocker medication reduces blood pressure and heart rate in response to activity and is used to treat angina and high blood pressure.

ACE inhibitors interfere with an enzyme in the blood called angiotensin. By blocking this enzyme the blood vessels are widened, which lowers blood pressure.

Statins work by reducing the amount of cholesterol that is made in the liver. Cholesterol contributes to the build-up of atheroma in the lining of the blood vessels.

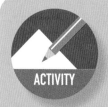

Activity 15.1

ACTIVITY

During the acute stages of an MI you may hear the team use the expression 'MONA'. Can you guess what this stands for? Remember, we need to treat the patient and make them comfortable.

Acid Reflux: H$_2$ Blockers

H$_2$ blockers are a group of medicines that reduce the amount of acid produced by the cells in the lining of the stomach. Their full name is histamine H$_2$ receptor antagonists. H$_2$ blockers may be prescribed to reduce acid reflux, promote healing of NSAID-associated ulcers (particularly duodenal ones) and treat ulcers in the stomach and duodenum.

The drugs prescribed may be:

- cimetidine,
- famotidine,
- nizatidine,
- ranitidine.

How Do They Work?

The stomach produces acid to help with the digestion of food. If the natural mucus barrier protecting the lining of the stomach against this corrosive acid has been broken down – perhaps due to taking NSAIDs – acid reflux may occur, irritating the oesophagus, which can cause heartburn and/or oesophagitis (that is, inflammation of the oesophagus). The letter H in this class of drugs stands for histamine. Histamine is a chemical produced by certain cells in the body, including cells found in the lining of the stomach. These cells are called enterochromaffin (ECL) cells. Histamine released by the ECL cells stimulates the parietal cells (which make acid) in the lining of the stomach to release acid. H$_2$ blockers stop the acid-making cells from responding to histamine, thus reducing the amount of acid produced by the stomach.

Possible Side Effects

The most common side effects from taking H$_2$ blockers are:

- Diarrhoea,
- Headache,
- Dizziness,
- Rash,
- Tiredness.

Most people taking these drugs, however, do not experience these side effects.

Drugs Used in a Cardiac Arrest Response

If you ever witness a cardiac arrest (in the hospital environment or in the middle of your local supermarket) you may wonder what the drugs are that are being gathered from the emergency drug box and resuscitation trolley or used by the paramedics. To be honest, it can be quite frightening, but remember that you will receive training in your basic life support classes and no one will expect you to lead the team! Let's look at the drugs and why they are given.

Adrenaline

This is the first drug administered in a cardiac arrest. Adrenaline strengthens cardiac contractions by stimulating the cardiac muscle, and it also concentrates the blood around the vital organs – especially the brain and the heart – by causing peripheral vasoconstriction. This combined effect increases the amount of blood circulating to the vital organs, and increases the chance of the heart returning to a normal rhythm. You may see adrenaline being administered every three to five minutes.

Amiodarone

After three attempts of unsuccessful electrical defibrillation amiodarone should be administered. It is given to treat specific cardiac arrhythmias (mainly ventricular fibrillation and ventricular tachycardia). It works by slowing down the metabolism of the cardiac tissue and also blocks the action of hormones that speed up the heart rate to produce a normal circulation.

Lidocaine

This drug is similar to amiodarone as it is used to treat specific cardiac arrhythmias by reducing the electrical activity of cardiac tissue. It can thus slow down a very fast heart rate. Lidocaine is not administered if amiodarone has already been given.

Atropine

This drug acts by blocking the effect of the vagus nerve on the heart. The vagus nerve normally slows the heart rate and during a cardiac arrest is a common cause of asystole. Atropine acts on the conduction system of the heart and accelerates the transmission of electrical impulses through the cardiac tissue. It is given to reverse asystole and severe bradycardia.

Additional Drugs

- Calcium chloride: calcium may improve weak or inefficient myocardial contractions when adrenaline has failed.
- Magnesium sulphate: magnesium is an important element in the contraction of muscular tissue, including cardiac muscle. A reduction in this electrolyte can frequently cause cardiac arrhythmias, resulting in cardiac arrest.

TEST YOUR KNOWLEDGE

1 What category of drugs does the NSAID aspirin belong to?
2 What is the antidote to paracetamol poisoning?
3 What does MAOI stand for?
4 Name four foods containing tyramine.
5 What are two of the active ingredients in co-codamol 8/500?
6 Name the drugs that may be used during a cardiac response.

KEY POINTS

- An overview of NSAIDs.
- An overview of paracetamol, MAOIs and the co-drugs.
- Looking at drugs used in specific medical conditions: stroke, post-MI, acid reflux, and during a cardiac arrest response.

WEB RESOURCES

BNF Adults: www.bnf.nice.org.uk
BNF Children: www.bnfc.nice.org.uk
Electronic Medicines Compendium: www.medicines.org.uk/emc

Chapter 16
. . . .
PAIN MANAGEMENT

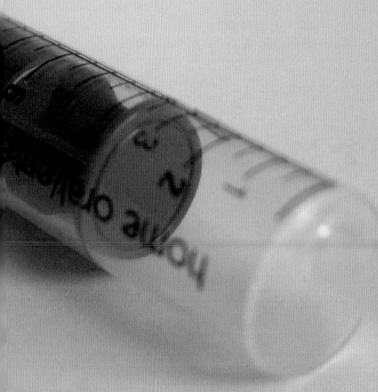

Medicine Management Skills for Nurses, Second Edition. Claire Boyd.
© 2022 John Wiley & Sons Ltd. Published 2022 by John Wiley & Sons Ltd.

LEARNING OUTCOMES

By the end of this chapter, you will have an understanding of the theory and practice of performing effective patient pain management.

Managing a patient's pain can be considered a clinical skill; at the very least it is good nursing practice. However, surveys conducted on patients who have been discharged from National Health Service (NHS) hospitals consistently tell us that approximately 87% of patients experience severe to moderate pain during their hospitalisation and that 42% of these patients then had to wait for their analgesia. Shocking!

Pain is often referred to as the fifth vital sign, meaning that as well as assessing the temperature, pulse, respirations, and blood pressure of a patient we need to monitor their pain levels and *act* on them. This applies not just in the acute hospital setting but also in primary and community care settings. This is due to the fact that statistics are telling us that almost 7.8 million people in the UK are living with chronic, intractable pain.

EFFECTS OF PAIN

When managed poorly, pain can have a devastating effect on the quality of life for those experiencing it, and for their families too. Acute and chronic pain are often associated with increased depression, anxiety, fear, and anger as well as impairments in memory, problem-solving, and information-processing speed.

The cost to society in the UK includes 4.6 million general practitioner (GP) appointments per year and £3.8 billion a year spent on incapacity benefit payments to those diagnosed with chronic pain. Pain is the second most common reason given by claimants of incapacity benefit.

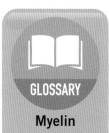

Myelin

Protein and phospholipid material covering axons of certain neurons, known as myelin sheaths.

NOW FOR THE SCIENCE BIT

Before we look at pain and its management in more detail, we first need to understand about the **pain pathways**. Pain is first detected by sensory nerve endings (receptors) known as **nociceptors**, which are found throughout the tissues of the body and carry impulses towards the central nervous system (CNS). Impulses are conducted via large, myelinated **A-delta fibres**, which conduct information at a fast rate, and/or by smaller **C fibres**, which conduct information at a slower rate due to their lack of myelination.

Tissue irritation or injury initiates the release of chemicals, such as prostaglandins, histamine, peptides, and kinins, that stimulate these nociceptors.

Once a receptor has been stimulated, it causes the nerve cell or neuron to 'fire' (become depolarised) and an action potential of electrical energy conveys a message along to a synapse, which is a gap between neurons. Neurotransmitters are the chemical messengers that cross this gap (for example, acetylcholine) and the neuron can continue to fire along one of three established pain pathways, as described here.

1   Dorsal column pathway: conveys information regarding pain localisation and vibration.
2   Spino-thalamic tract pathway: conveys information of the pain site and the pain's intensity.
3   Spino-recticular tract pathway: involved within the limbic system, which is responsible for feelings and emotions.

These ascending pain pathways stimulate areas of the brain. This explains the subjectivity of pain perception due to the incorporation of physiological, social and psychological elements of the pain experience, and why anxiety often makes pain worse.

PAIN GATE THEORY

We can see then that pain perception is a complex process: Melzack and Wall attempted to explain this complexity and variability with the development of the Gate Control Theory way back in 1965 (today more commonly known as the pain gate theory).

According to this theory, a painful stimulus can be modified by a gating mechanism situated in the substantia gelatinosa in the dorsal horn of the spinal cord. The theory proposes that it is possible to alter the transmission of pain by deliberately activating another type of sensory receptor to dampen the pain perception; for example, by a patient rubbing her arm after a subcutaneous injection. Therefore, by rubbing the painful spot, the rubbing signals get through and block the pain signals. In other words we can 'close the gate' or block the pain.

CLASSIFICATIONS OF PAIN

Pain can be classified according to how long it has lasted and what is happening in the nervous system. There are many different types of pain, four of which are:

1   Acute pain,
2   Chronic pain,
3   Nociceptive pain,
4   Neuropathic pain.

In most cases pain is an acute, short-lasting event, such as a throb, dull ache, or even a sharp, piercing soreness.

Acute pain is accompanied by signs of hyperactivity in the autonomic nervous system, such as sweating and vasoconstriction. We can often observe these symptoms in patients who are in pain.

But for some people pain may be longer lasting. This is referred to as **chronic pain** and may never go away. Chronic pain can severely affect one's life, 'making every waking moment a misery' as one patient described to me. The term chronic pain is often used to refer to pain that lasts for more than six weeks (although some literature states this to be three months) and can be unbearable, making everyday activities difficult or impossible to manage. Chronic pain is often more difficult to treat as it produces changes in the CNS, leading to changes in the autonomic nervous system, known as **adaption**. The patient may not show many outward signs that they actually have any pain. Many inexperienced health carers may then doubt the pain even exists in the individual. Chronic pain often produces changes in personality, life style, and activities of living.

Neuropathic pain does not require a stimulus, but can be caused due to damage to the nervous system, and is often described as 'electrical', 'tingling', or 'pins and needles'.

Nociceptive pain is a response to an obvious stimulus, such as burning, cutting, broken bones, or sprains. It can be described as 'deep', 'squeezing', and 'dull' in origin. It may be accompanied by nausea and vomiting.

ASSESSMENT OF PAIN

A pain scale measures a patient's pain intensity and there are many examples of pain scales used in health care. Many acute-pain assessment documents have a built-in scale, such as the chart used for adults shown in Figure 16.1.

Here we can see that the intensity of the pain is graded from 0 to 3:

0   No pain,
1   No pain at rest, mild on movement,
2   Intermittent pain at rest, moderate on movement,
3   Severe pain.

Other numerical rating scales use 1–10, with 0 being 'no pain' and 10 representing the 'worst possible pain'. In childcare, the Wong–Baker FACES Pain Rating Scale is often used, which is recommended for children aged 3 and above. This is a set of faces going from 'no hurt' (a smiling face) to 'hurts worst' (a sad, often crying face). In neonates and infants, observational parameters may be used.

Nausea and sedation are often also assessed in conjunction with pain, due to the analgesic effect

Adult Acute Pain Observation Chart

North Bristol **NHS**
NHS Trust

Frequency of obs.
(eg. ¼ hrly,
½ hrly, 1 hrly)

(insert frequency, date and time)

Patient details:

Name
DoB
ID number
Ward
Date
Consultant

Patient sticker here

PRESCRIBED DRUG

TICK INFUSION METHOD   PCA ☐   EPIDURAL ☐   NERVE BLOCK/INFUSION ☐   PCEA ☐

Date:	Time:																			
Time:																				

PAIN SCORE																					
Rest: R	3																				
Movement: M	2																				
Both: X	1																				
	0																				

Sedation Score: 0/1/2/3																				
Respiratory Rate: 1 min.																				
Nausea Score: 0/N/V																				

PCA / PCEA
Total Demands:																				
Demands Given:																				
Background Infusion																				
Rate ml/hr:																				
mls in syringe/bag:																				
mls given:																				
Total infused mls:																				
Bolus mls:																				
Total given:																				
Check Site																				

EPIDURAL/ORTHOPAEDIC (PEDAL CHECKS)
Pulse	R																				
	L																				
Warmth	R																				
	L																				
Colour	R																				
	L																				
Sensation	R																				
	L																				
Movement	R																				
	L																				

North Bristol NHS Trust Pain Service 2008   RVJ0700 (LGD)

Figure 16.1 Adult acute pain observation chart. Source: Permission to reproduce this image is granted by North Bristol NHS Trust and University Hospitals Bristol NHS Foundation Trust.

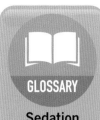

GLOSSARY

Sedation

A restful state of mind, usually brought about by the use of drugs, known as sedatives.

of the pain-management therapy. A patient's pain management may cause them to experience nausea and increased levels of sedation, as many of these drugs have this unfortunate side effect. We would need to tweak the analgesia so that these effects are limited, but not so much that they start to experience higher levels of pain.

It is for this reason that patients with opiate infusions are often observed every 15 minutes for the first 2 hours and then every 30 minutes for the following 2 hours. From then onwards, observations may commence every 2 hours, depending on the patient's condition. The respiratory rate, sedation score, and pump readings are recorded hourly until the infusion has ceased. Patients on opiates from other routes are usually observed hourly for pain levels, respiratory rate (counted over one full minute), and sedation levels, in addition to their other routine observations. We can see from the above chart that the sedation score goes from 0 to 3.

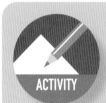

Activity 16.1

ACTIVITY

What do you think 0, 1, 2, and 3 represent with respect to Sedation score on the pain observation chart? If you saw S on this chart, what do you think it might mean?

0 =
1 =
2 =
3 =
S =

As well as the actual scale of pain, in order to manage pain effectively healthcare professionals will need to gather further information as part of a pain assessment, by asking questions such as:

- Where is the pain?
- When did it start?
- What makes it worse?
- What helps to ease it?
- Is it a sharp pain or dull, aching, throbbing, shooting, or burning pain?

STRATEGIES TO MANAGE PAIN

Years ago pain management was often managed in only one way: the medical approach to care, using prescription medicines only. Many hospitals now have pain clinics to help patients to manage their pain, offering many alternative techniques to go with the more traditional approach. This is referred to as the complimentary approach and includes treatments such as:

- Acupuncture,
- Osteopathy,
- Deep-breathing exercises,
- Massage,
- Tai chi,
- Yoga,
- Relaxation,
- Botulinum toxin injections (for muscle spasms).

Many pain-management strategies combine more than one approach, for example medication and relaxation therapies.

ANALGESIC LADDER

Analgesics, often referred to as 'painkillers' by our patients, are groups of drugs used to treat pain. The World Health Organization devised the WHO Analgesic Ladder to assist health carers in managing pain, tailored to a person's individual needs.

The ladder takes a stepped approach to the use of analgesics according to their group or category – such as simple analgesics – which can be seen below:

- Simple analgesics: paracetamol and non-steroidal anti-inflammatory drugs (NSAIDs),
- Weak opioids: tramadol, codeine,
- Strong opioids: morphine, fentanyl, oxycodone, pethidine,
- Adjuvants: these drugs were not originally for pain, but they have been found to be effective in difficult-to-manage pain. They include antidepressants and anticonvulsants.

The national discussion forum and community for UK healthcare professionals (www.pain-talk.co.uk) devised a recommended analgesia ladder (Figure 16.2) for adult patients, which was based on the WHO Analgesic Ladder.

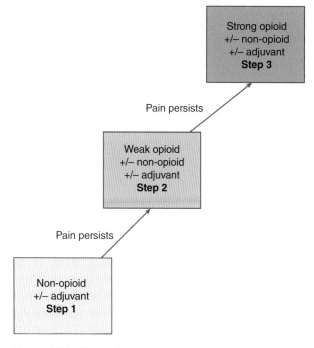

Figure 16.2 The analgesic ladder. Source: From Lister, Hofland, and Graton. (2020).

Step 1 relates to a pain score of 1, equating to mild pain; step 2 relates to a pain score of 2, equating to moderate pain; and step 3 relates to a pain score of 3, equating to severe pain.

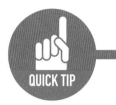

QUICK TIP

Opiates are derived directly from the juice of the opium poppy, e.g. morphine. *Opioids* include all naturally occurring opiates and also include synthetic drugs with opiate-like or morphine-like qualities, e.g. tramadol.

So, Tramadol is an opioid. Morphine is an opiate and also an opioid.

MORPHINE

As we can see from the analgesic ladder, the most severe pain may require morphine and it is important to have an understanding of this medication. First, morphine is the 'gold standard' for all opiates. It can be prescribed in a variety of ways:

Intramuscular injection: e.g. 10 mg morphine intramuscular (IM) hourly *pro re nata* (PRN),

Oramorph: e.g. 10–20 mg Oramorph two hourly PRN,

Intravenous injection: intravenous (IV) morphine up to 10 mg in incremental doses (1–2 mg per dose); this is written under STAT prescriptions on the drug chart and titrated to the patient's condition.

Correct Dilution for IV Morphine

- Add 10 mg of morphine (1 ml) to 9 ml of saline 0.9% in a 10 ml syringe.
- This equals 10 ml in total in the syringe.
- Each millilitre then contains 1 mg of morphine.
- Give 2 mg (2 ml) and wait for five minutes.
- Judge the effect (pain assessment), give a further 2 mg if necessary and repeat as necessary.

Complications/Side Effects of Opiates

- Pain
- Over-sedation
- Respiratory depression
- Nausea and vomiting
- Constipation
- Pruritus (itching)
- Hallucinations

Observations

- Pain level
- Sedation level
- Respiratory rate and oxygen saturation
- Blood pressure and heart rate
- Incidence of nausea and vomiting

Observe the patient continuously during administration. It is important to *stay with the patient.* Document your observations every 15 minutes. Continue to observe and document all observations for at least 30 minutes following the last dose of morphine.

Antidote to Most Opiates

- Naloxone 400 µg/ml.
- Dilute 1 ml in 3 ml of saline 0.9%.
- This equals 4 ml in total.
- Each millilitre now contains 100 µg of naloxone.
- Give in incremental doses of 100 µg (1 ml) and wait for five minutes.
- Repeat as necessary and titrate to effect.

Predictors of Dose

- In children: weight
- In adults: weight plus age

Care must be taken with anyone over the age of 70.

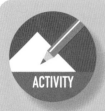

Activity 16.2

Why must care be taken with anyone over the age of 70 when giving morphine?

BALANCED ANALGESIA

When administering opiates, give:

* Regular paracetamol,

plus

* A regular NSAID.

Why is Paracetamol Usually Prescribed with Morphine?

Well, paracetamol (or acetaminophen) has a 'morphine-sparing effect' and is used to 'pull out' the analgesic effect in order to reduce the total amount of morphine required.

NSAIDs can also be a useful adjuvant to narcotic analgesia, enhancing the activity of narcotics, especially because they possess anti-inflammatory properties. NSAIDs are less effective as an analgesic in non-inflamed tissues.

PALLIATIVE CARE

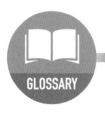

Palliative care
Care for patients whose condition is described as terminal.

Palliative medicine
Medicine that gives temporary relief from the symptoms of a disease but which does not actually cure the condition.

Patients in palliative care may require a device known as a syringe driver to let them receive drugs at a constant rate to maintain comfort and symptom relief. Indications for use are:

- Terminally ill patients,
- Patients who may be experiencing persistent nausea and vomiting,
- Patients who are unable to swallow oral medications,
- Unconscious patients,
- Patients experiencing extreme weakness and/or who have poor alimentary absorption.

These devices can deliver the medication in the syringe over a period of 1 or 24 hours. The medication is drawn up into a syringe, mixed with an infusate (water for injection) and then set into the syringe driver pump. The other end of the syringe has an infusion line with a small needle at the end that is attached to the patient's body site to let them receive the medication. Sites used may be the:

- Anterior aspect of the upper arms,
- Anterior chest wall,
- Anterior aspect of the thighs,
- Anterior abdominal wall.

Setting up a syringe driver is a specialised skill that requires training, but as a student nurse there is nothing to stop you watching this being done by qualified nurses and learning the procedure if you come across such devices.

Monitoring of these devices is usually conducted every four hours in a hospital setting and on every visit in the community. It is important to check that the correct amount of fluid has been delivered within the expected time frame and that symptom control is being maintained.

With a syringe driver two or three different drugs may be mixed together in one syringe, such as anti-emetics and pain relief. However, some drugs are incompatible together, such as cyclizine and hyoscine butylbromide (e.g. Buscopan). The palliative care team will be able to advise nurses about drug compatibility. Drugs commonly used in syringe drivers can be seen in Table 16.1.

Table 16.1 Drugs commonly used in syringe drivers.

Name of drug	Indications	Usual dose range over 24 h
Diamorphine	Pain	Starting dose of 5–10 mg, then titrate to patient's needs
Cyclizine	Nausea/vomiting	100–150 mg
Metoclopramide	Nausea/vomiting	30–60 mg
Haloperidol	Nausea/vomiting	1.5–5 mg (nausea and vomiting)
	Agitation	5–10 mg (agitation)
Levomepromazine	Nausea/vomiting	5–25 mg (nausea and vomiting)
	Agitation	25–100 mg (agitation)
Midazolam	Agitation	10–100 mg
	Respiratory panic	10–20 mg (agitation)
	Severe anxiety	20–30 mg (anti-convulsant)
	Convulsions	
Hyoscine butylbromide	Helps dry bronchial secretions/death rattle Reduces bowel colic	40–120 mg
Hyoscine hydrobromide	Helps dry bronchial secretions/death rattle Reduces bowel colic	0.8–2.4 mg
Glycopyrronium	Helps dry bronchial secretions/death rattle	0.8–2.4 mg

NOTE: check your own area's protocol, as amounts may vary.

TEST YOUR KNOWLEDGE

Case Study

Yvonne Baker fell down the stairs one night while sleepwalking and was woken – along with the whole street – by the pain of a broken tibia and fibula. Yvonne also had a small laceration to her right arm, which was bleeding.

1   What type of pain did Yvonne experience in her right arm?

She was taken to hospital for surgery for a very complex break and underwent metal fixation. She was found to have nerve damage to her leg. Since the bones have healed Yvonne walks with a walking stick and experiences constant pain in her leg with very restricted mobility.

2   Why is Yvonne prescribed anti-depressants to go with her analgesics, even though she does not feel depressed?

Yvonne describes her pain as 'like hot electrical shocks' going up her leg, which she describes as 'unbearable'.

3   What type of pain is Yvonne now experiencing?

During these episodes of pain, Yvonne's husband notices that she pulls out the hairs in her eyebrows, to 'help the pain'. He thinks she has gone mad, but there is a reason for this.

4   What theory of pain can explain what Yvonne is doing to control her pain?

At work Yvonne gets on with her day-to-day tasks, so much so that her work colleagues doubt she is even in pain. This is because Yvonne shows no outward signs of pain.

5   What is this called?

Yvonne has been advised by the Pain Clinic in her local hospital to try relaxation therapy, as she has noticed that when she is anxious the pain experience is worse.

6   Could this therapy work for her?

KEY POINTS

- Effects of pain on the individual and on society.
- The pain pathways and the pain gate theory.
- The classifications of pain.
- Documentation for pain assessment.
- Pain-management strategies.
- The analgesic ladder.

WEB RESOURCES

BNF Adults: www.bnf.nice.org.uk
BNF Children: www.bnfc.nice.org.uk
Pain: www.paincoalition.org.uk
Pain: www.pain-talk.co.uk
WHO: www.who.int
WHO Pain Ladder: www.who.int/cancer/palliative/
   painladder/en/

REFERENCES

Lister, S., Hofland, J., and Graton, H. (eds.) (2020). *The Royal Marsden of Clinical Nursing Procedures*, 10e. Wiley.

Chapter 17
. . . .
CASE STUDY

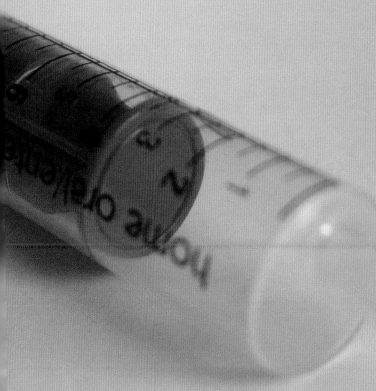

LEARNING OUTCOMES

By the end of this chapter, you will have an understanding of medications administered for medical conditions and their possible side-effects, as well as learning about how cultural issues have a bearing on medication. Lastly you will learn to be patient with staff new to healthcare.

We all started from scratch when embarking on our health-care career, be that as a Registered Nurse, Midwife, Nursing Associate, Assistant Practitioner, etc. and can remember what a difference some kind colleague in the workplace made to our shift. Now you have read the previous chapters, lets start putting some of our knowledge into practice.

Stephen is a student nurse who will complete his placement, at the end of todays shift on the Acute Medical Unit at a large National Health Service (NHS) Trust. Everyday Stephen takes notes for his own understanding. Sarah is a Nursing Associate who is just starting her placement on the unit today, and is very keen. Stephen has given her his notes, on medications, for today's admitted patients, hoping to build her knowledge.

NOTES ON PATIENTS' MEDICAL CONDITIONS, MEDICATION, AND POSSIBLE SIDE-EFFECTS

Patients medical condition	Drug examples	Possible side-effects
Acute Diarrhoea	Loperamide – 2 mg PO Administer after loose stool	Nausea Flatulence Gastrointestinal (GI) discomfort
Alcohol detoxification	Diazepam – 200 mg PO (Maximum dose 200 mg)	Drowsiness Light-headedness confusion

Patients medical condition	Drug examples	Possible side-effects
Anaemia (Iron deficiency)	Ferrous fumarate – 200 mg PO	Dizziness GI disturbances
Angina	Glyceryl tri-nitrate (GTN) SL Spray	Postural hypotension Dizziness
Yeast Infection – thrush (Vaginal candidiasis)	Clotrimazole – 200 mg pessary for three nights PV	Local irritation May damage latex condoms and diaphragms
Cardiac arrhythmias	Digoxin – 62.5 µg PO Do not administer if HR < 60	Nausea Diarrhoea Xanthopsia (yellowing of the eyesight)
Deep Vein Thrombosis	Warfarin sodium – 3 mg PO Daily international normalized ratio (INR) blood tests	Increased bruising and risk of bleeding
Stroke	Aspirin – 75 mg PO (non-steroidal anti-inflammatory drug [NSAID])	Gastric irritation Stomach ulcers
Schizophrenia	Clozapine – 200 mg PO am 500 mg – nocte	Photosensitisation drowsiness
Acute anxiety	Zopiclone – 75 mg	Nausea Headache dizziness
Rheumatoid arthritis	Prednisone – 20 mg MR PO	Fluid-retention causing swollen feet and ankles Headache Feeling tired
Constipation and bowel cleansing (for investigation procedure)	Docusate sodium – 120 mg PR	Abdominal cramp Rash
Depression	Citalopram – 20 mg	GI reaction Weight loss

Patients medical condition	Drug examples	Possible side-effects
Insulin Dependant Diabetes Mellitus (IDDM)	Metformin – 500 mg *ter die sumendus* (TDS) Monitor blood glucose (BG) Levels	GI side-effects Nausea Vomiting
Fluid Retention – Diuretics	Furosemide – 40 mg Maintain Fluid chart	Polyuria – excessive passing of urine Postural hypotension Hypokalaemia (low potassium)
Dyspepsia (indigestion/ heartburn)	Omeprazole EC – 20 mg PO	GI disturbance Headache
Epilepsy – tonic-clonic seizures	Phenytoin – 30 mg/5 ml PO Oral Suspension	Acne Nausea Diarrhoea
Heart failure	Lisinopril – 2.5 mg PO	Hypotension Dizziness
Hypertension	Atenolol – 50 mg PO	Hypotension Dizziness
Chest Infection – bacterial	Amoxicillin – 500 mg PO *Quater die sumendus* (QDS)	Nausea Vomiting
Migraine	Rizatriptan – 10 mg SL wafer PRN	Alertness decreased Asthenia (abnormal physical weakness or lack of energy)
Gout	Allopurinol – 200 mg PO PC (after food)	Hypersensitivity reactions Rash
Nausea and vomiting	Metoclopramide – 10 mg TDS Dose titrated to patient's weight	Drowsiness Diarrhoea Restlessness
Pyrexia	Paracetamol – 500 mg PO QDS	Rare Malaise
Pain – auto-immune disorder	Naproxen – 250 mg PO QDS (NSAID) PC (after food)	Gastric irritation

Patients medical condition	Drug examples	Possible side-effects
Contraception	Microgynon 30 (Ethinylestradiol 30 µg levonorgestrel 150 µg combined) – 1 tablet PO	Nausea Vomiting Thromboembolic and liver disease
Pain – post procedure	Morphine – MST – 10 mg PO QDS Opioid	Nausea Vomiting constipation
Parkinsons disease	Levodopa + benserazide/ carbidopa/entacapone MR 1 tablet (max 10 tablets per day)	Nausea Anorexia 'on-off' effect
Asthma	Salbutamol – 100 µg Pressurised device – 2 doses IHL PRN	Oral yeast infection
Smoking cessation	Nicotine – 7 mg per 24 h Transdermal patch × 1	Bloating Constipation Dry mouth
Thyroid condition – hypothyroidism	Levothyroxine – 50 µg PO	Dosing excess: Tachycardia Arrhythmia insomnia
Eczema	Hydrocortisone 0.5% cream 2 fingertip unit (FTU)'s on affected area Spread Thinly BD	Thinning of the skin Irritation of the skin Increased hair growth
Pernicious anaemia	Hydroxocobalamin 1 mg every 3 mo IM Vit. B12	Dizziness Headache Pruritus
Osteoporosis (Calcium deficiency)	Calcium carbonate 1 tablet OD By mouth do not swallow (chew)	Constipation Flatulence Nausea
Dehydration	1 l Sodium Chloride 0.9% Over 8 h IV Maintain Fluid Chart	Hypervolemia (excess fluids) Hypernatremia (high levels of sodium) Access site infection

TEST YOUR KNOWLEDGE

17.1 Sarah is very grateful to Stephen for his help, but looking at his sheet, she has written down a few queries she has! As Stephen has fainted, can you answer her questions?

Query

1   What is GI discomfort?
2   What does PO mean?
3   What does GTN – SL mean?
4   What is PV?
5   What is a daily INR test?
6   What is a NSAID?
7   What does Nocte mean?
8   What is a MR tablet?
9   What does PR mean?
10 What does 'monitor BG levels' mean?
11 What does IDDM mean?
12 Why does a fluid chart need to be maintained for the patient prescribed Furosemide?
13 What does EC mean?
14 What is a SL wafer?
15 What does PC stand for?
16 What does titrate to patient's weight mean?
17 What does QDS mean?
18 What is a transdermal patch?
19 What is a FTU measurement?
20 What does BD stand for?
21 What does IM mean?
22 What does OD stand for?
23 Can you swallow the drug that states 'to chew'?

17.2 Stephen tells Sarah that he has obtained some information about the UK's ten most prescribed generic drugs overall:

1	Simvastatin	37.3 million
2	Aspirin	33.9 million
3	Levothyroxine Sodium	21.9 million
4	Ramipril	19.3 million
5	Bendroflumethiazide	18.8 million

6	Paracetamol	18.8 million
7	Salbutamol	18.7 million
8	Omeprazole	18.3 million Proton-pump inhibitors
9	Lansoprazole	14.9 million Proton-pump inhibitors
10	Co-codamol	14.6 million

Source: NHS Information Centre

Stephen tells Sarah that drugs for cardiovascular disease (CVD) make up four of the top five places among the top ten most prescribed generic drugs. The thyroid drug Levothyroxine Sodium is the only non-CVD treatment in the top five.

Which of these drugs have Stephen and Sarah seen on today's admissions to the unit?

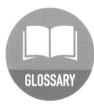

GLOSSARY

CVD = Heart and Circulatory Disease, known as cardiovascular disease (CVD) and causes a quarter of all deaths in the UK.

17.3 Living in a multi-cultural country, it is important that healthcare professionals are fully aware of all relevant aspects of different cultures and the effects that they have on their medications.

Religion	Religious fact	Issues to consider
Buddhism	During the religious festival of Wesak, believers should 'refrain from taking substantial food after midday' (from noon to dawn).	A Client requires aspirin TDS, as prepared in his blister pack. How will this religious fact affect his medication administration?
Christianity	During the religious festival of Lent, many believers undertake observance of self-denial and commit to fasting or giving up certain luxuries as a form of penitence.	Could a medication administered to 'reduce pain' be considered as a luxury?

Religion	Religious fact	Issues to consider
Hinduism	Most Hindus do not eat beef and/or pork and adhere to strict vegetarianism. The cow is the most revered animal for Hindus.	A client has been prescribed a capsule, which you have read in the Patient Information leaflet 'contains gelatine' – is this a problem/can the client still take this medication?
Islam	Followers of Islam are called Muslims. During Ramadan, Muslims can eat and drink as long as the sun has set. Exempt from taking part in the Ramadan fast are: Children, the sick, the elderly, the mentally handicapped, and anyone putting their health at serious risk by fasting, pregnant women, and those on a tiring journey.	You notice that your client has 'cc' written on a bottle of medication sitting on the mantelpiece in their front room. Is this a problem for your Muslim client presently fasting?
Judaism	Passover is one of the most important festivals in the Jewish year. Four small glasses of wine are drunk during these celebrations in order to symbolise 'joy and happiness'.	Your client is taking a medication called Phenytoin for their epilepsy – do you have any concerns?
Sikhism	Sikhism followers adhere to a system of Langar (or communal kitchen) – to demonstrate the need to share and have equally between all people.	Your client has popped out two of her prescribed cardiac pills from her blister pack to give to her sister, whom she states is experiencing 'flutters to her heart also'. Do you have any concerns about this?

KEY POINTS

- Looking at patients' medical conditions and drugs administered for these and their potential side-effects.
- How religious considerations may need to be addressed when administering medications.
- Being kind and helpful to those following in our healthcare footsteps.

WEB RESOURCES

British National Formulary: www.bnf.org

NHS Information Centre: www.england.nhs.uk/publication/ nhs-england-drugs-list

Medicines and Healthcare Products Regulatory Agency: www.mhra.gov.uk/government/organisation/ medicines-and-healthcare

Chapter 18
· ·
KNOWLEDGE TEST

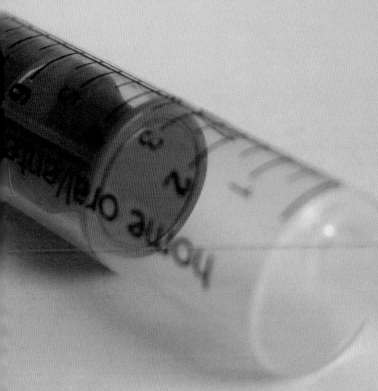

Medicine Management Skills for Nurses, Second Edition. Claire Boyd.
© 2022 John Wiley & Sons Ltd. Published 2022 by John Wiley & Sons Ltd.

LEARNING OUTCOMES

This chapter will give you the opportunity to demonstrate your understanding of the procedures and principles of medicines management.

To help increase your medicines-management knowledge, and to put everything together that you have read and learned about in this book, see if you can answer these questions.

1　What is the medication process chain?
2　When administering medication, what are the five rights that we should adhere to?
3　What is the parenteral route of drug administration?
4　What is said to be the percentage bioavailability of drugs administered by the IV route?
5　What does the word pharmacodynamics mean?
6　What does the word pharmacokinetics mean?
7　What is a drug interaction?
8　What is the drug acetaminophen more commonly known as?
9　What is an adverse drug reaction (ADR)?
10　What is pharmacovigilance?
11　What is the name of the document that needs to be completed to report an adverse drug reaction?
12　What is a PIL?
　　Go and make a cup of tea and have a biscuit. Ready for some more?
13　Categories of medicine: what is a GSL?
14　Categories of medicine: what is a POM?
15　You see 1 TDS on a bottle of pills: state many and how often should you take this medication.
16　You saw CC on a bottle of pills: what does it mean?
17　What is a depot injection?
18　In regard to the storage of medicines, what is the cold chain?
19　Name the three classes of drugs listed in the Misuse of Drugs Act, 1971.

20 What is a proprietary drug name?

21 What is the proprietary name for salbutamol (albuterol)?

22 What does the abbreviation BNF mean?

23 Where should sublingual medication be placed on/in the body?Want to carry on? Go on, you're on a roll now!

24 What does it mean for a medication to have an enteric coating?

25 Can you state what some of the possible side effects might be to these commonly prescribed drugs?

Analgesics containing codeine
Antidepressants, antiparkinsonian drugs
Antibiotic allergy, non-steroidal anti-inflammatory drugs (NSAIDs)
Blood-pressure medication
Sleeping tablets, sedatives

26 A patient requires 225 mg of ranitidine orally. In the ward are 150 mg tablets. How many tablets should be given?

27 A patient needs 750 mg of penicillin. On hand are tablets of strength 250 mg. How many tablets should be given?

28 A patient is prescribed 15 mg of codeine phosphate. Stock on hand is 30 mg codeine phosphate tablets. How many tablets should the patient receive?

29 A patient is prescribed 150 mg of soluble aspirin. On hand are 300 mg tablets. What number of tablets should be given?

30 Amoxicillin is presented as 500 mg per ampoule. It is diluted to a volume of 10 ml. Your patient is prescribed 1 g. What volume of amoxicillin do you draw up for injection?

31 IV digoxin comes as 500 µg in 2 ml. The prescription is to administer 300 µg of digoxin. What volume of digoxin you would administer?

32 Vancomycin is presented as a 1 g ampoule. It is diluted to a volume of 20 ml. Your patient is prescribed 750 mg. What volume of vancomycin do you draw up for injection?

33 What is a depot injection?

Have a break now and do some more tomorrow. Remember – You don't have to complete these questions all in one sitting!

34 Explain the intramuscular injection route.
35 What is the Z-track technique for intramuscular injections?
36 Explain the subcutaneous injection route.
37 Explain the intravenous injection route.
38 Explain the intradermal injection route.
39 What is a needle bevel?
40 If a drug is presented in micrograms, how is this abbreviated on the prescription chart?

Can you do the calculations for the following prescriptions?

41 Prescribed: 80 mg erythromycin; stock ampoule: 100 mg/2 ml
42 Prescribed: 60 mg pethidine; stock ampoule: 100 mg/2 ml
43 Prescribed: 15 mg omnopon; stock ampoule: 20 mg/ml
44 Prescribed: 60 mg cortisone; stock ampoule: 125 mg/5 ml
45 Prescribed: 500 mg streptomycin; stock ampoule: 1 g in 3 ml
46 Prescribed: 150 µg digoxin; stock ampoule: 500 µg in 2 ml
47 Prescribed: 15 000 units calciparine; stock ampoule: 25 000 units in 1 ml
48 Prescribed: 7 mg/h isoket; stock ampoule: 500 µg/ml
49 Prescribed: 50 mg gentamicin; stock ampoule: 80 mg/2 ml
50 Prescribed: 50 mg/min phenytoin; stock ampoule: 1 g/100 ml

Well we did go on a bit here: time for a break?

51 Calculate the drip rate to the nearest whole drop: 420 ml of blood is to be given to a patient over 4 hours using a blood administration set (15 drops per ml).

52 Calculate the drip rate to the nearest whole drop: 500 ml of sodium chloride 0.9% over 4 hours with a standard giving set.

53 Calculate the drip rate to the nearest whole drop: 50 ml of Hartmann's solution is to be given to a child over 1 hour. Calculate the rate in drops per minute using a paediatric/microdrip giving set (60 drops per ml)

54 Calculate the drip rate to the nearest whole drop: glucose infusion, 500 ml, over 6 hours. Standard giving set.

55 Calculate the drip rate to the nearest whole drop: a child is to have sodium chloride 0.45% with glucose 2.5% at 400 ml over 12 hours. Calculate the rate using a microdrop giving set.

56 Calculate the drip rate to the nearest whole drop: 500 ml of Haemaccel is to run over 1 hour.

57 What is the name of the stool assessment chart?

58 What does the abbreviation DRE mean in relation to bowel care?

59 What does the abbreviation AF mean?

60 How would you administer a vaginal pessary?

Put the kettle on: time for a break!

61 How do you measure a fingertip unit?

62 What is the procedure for applying ear drops to a patient or service user?

63 If I saw PRN on a prescription chart how often would I be required to administer this medicine?

64 List three of the common mistakes made when administering inhaler medications.

65 What is a preventer inhaler?

66 A drug is to be administered IV over 24 hours. What is this called?

67 What is an isotonic crystalloid?

68 Are blood products isotonic, hypotonic, or hypertonic?

69 What is the normal physiological range of the electrolyte sodium?

70 What is speed shock?

71 What is free flow?

Let's break here and start again tomorrow.

72 Name four advantages of intravenous bolus injections.

73 Describe what displacement means.

74 A patient is prescribed 125 mg of amoxicillin from a 250 mg vial. The displacement value for amoxicillin 250 mg is 0.2 ml. You are required to make up a total volume of 5 ml with water for injection. How much fluid do you add?

75 What is the name for fluids or medicines that are administered over 24 hours via the IV route?

76 Name four advantages of the continuous intravenous infusion route.

77 What is the formula for working out the intravenous infusion rate in millilitres per hour?

78 An insulin infusion containing 50 units of human Actrapid has been diluted with 50 ml of sodium chloride, which has been running at:

4.5 ml/h for 3 hours
3 ml/h for 1 hour
2 ml/h for 1 hour
4 ml/h for 2 hours

How many units of Actrapid insulin in total has the patient received?

79 What is a PEG an abbreviation for?

80 What is a PEJ an abbreviation for?

81 What is a NG an abbreviation for?

82 A patient is on an enteral feeding regime. What methods are there for administering it?

Had enough? Let's do some more tomorrow.

83 What is NSAIDs short for?

84 Name one side effects of taking the drug aspirin.

85 What is MAOI short for?

86 What are the foods to be avoided by an individual taking a MAOI medication?

87   What are the active ingredients in the drug co-amilofruse 2.5/20?

88   What are the active ingredients in the drug co-amoxiclav 250/125?

89   What are the four most common drugs that a patient who has previously experienced a myocardial infarction is likely to be prescribed and why?

90   Let's look at some dosages according to body weight: a patient weighing 70 kg is prescribed 10 mg/kg/h of a drug. How many milligrams per hour of the drug does the patient need?

91   Paracetamol is prescribed as 10 mg/kg and can be given 8-hourly. How much would you give to a baby weighing 2.5 kg?

92   Ranitidine is prescribed as 2 mg/kg. How many milligrams will be prescribed to a baby weighing 0.570 kg?

93   A child weighs 12 kg. Calculate the single dose needed for the prescribed erythromycin 40 mg/kg/d, four doses per day.

94   A child weighs 36 kg. Calculate a single dose of flucloxacillin 100 mg/kg/d, four doses per day.

95   A child weighs 27 kg. Calculate a single dose of ampicillin 80 mg/kg/d, four doses per day.

Have a copy of the BNF to hand. . .

96   What is gentamicin? What are the indications, for use?

97   What is ibuprofen? What are the indications, for use?

98   What is gliclazide? What are the indications, for use?

99   What is dexamethasone? What are the indications, for use?

100   What is Flupentixol? What are its indications, for use?

Done!

Answers to Activities, Questions, and 'Test Your Knowledge'

Activity 1.1

STAT	immediately
AC	*ante cibum* (before food)
BD	*bis die* (twice daily)
OD	*omni die* (every day)
OM	*omni mane* (every morning)
ON	*omni nocte* (every night)
PC	*post cibum* (after food)
PRN	*pro re nata* (when required)
QDS	*quater die sumendus* (to be taken four times daily)
QQH	*quarta quaque hora* (every 4 hours)
TDS	*ter die sumendus* (to be taken three times daily)
TID	*Ter in die* (three times daily)

Activity 1.2

AF = Atrial fibrillation

DKA = Diabetic ketoacidosis

INR = International normalized ratio (clotting factor)

BNF = British national formulary

DM = Diabetes mellitus

MAOI = Monoamine oxidase inhibitor

BP = Blood pressure

DVT = Deep vein thrombosis

MHRA = Medicines and Healthcare Products

CHD = Coronary heart disease

GI = Gastrointestinal

MI = Myocardial infarction

COPD = Chronic obstructive pulmonary disease

GTN = Glyceryl trinitrate

NG = Nasogastric

Medicine Management Skills for Nurses, Second Edition. Claire Boyd.

CR = Controlled release

DH = Department of Health

NPSA = National Patient Safety Agency

NSAID = Non-steroidal anti-inflammatory drug

PPI = Proton pump inhibitor

IDDM = Insulin-dependent diabetes mellitus

NMC = Nursing and Midwifery Council (includes nursing associates)

OTC = Over the counter

WHO = World Health Organisation

GP = General practitioner (Doctor)

NHS = National Health Service

NICE = National Institute for Health and Care Excellence

NIDDM = Non-insulin-dependent-diabetes-mellitus

PEG = Percutaneous endoscopic gastrosyomy

CD = Controlled drug

Activity 1.3

1. ITH — intrathecal
2. SC — subcutaneous
3. ID — intradermal
4. IV — intravenous
5. IM — intramuscular
6. O — oral
7. INH — inhalation
8. NEB — nebulisation
9. TOP — topical

Activity 1.4

1. Weight (kg) × dose 70 kg × 10 mg = 700 mg/h

2. 5 g = 5000 mg. Therefore, there are 5000 mg in 500 ml. The hourly rate is:

   Volume of drug to be given =

   $$\frac{\text{what you want}}{\text{what you've got}} \times \text{volume}$$

   $$\frac{700mg/h}{5000mg} \times 500mL = 70mL/h$$

Chapter 1 Questions

1.1 No. Use your professional judgement and omit this medication if safe to do so (i.e. after discussion with medical staff). You will need to document that the drug was omitted on the prescription chart, giving the reason why.

1.2 A near miss is a medication error that does not result in patient harm. Example: a dose of 500 mg amoxycillin is prepared instead of 250 mg, but corrected before reaching the patient.

1.3 Try to cover up your mistake. You must report it. Admit your error to the patient.

1.4 Another high-risk group is the elderly. They make up 18% of the population, and receive 45% of all prescribed drugs, so therefore are most susceptible to adverse drug reactions and drug interactions. Drugs such as morphine are metabolised more slowly by the elderly, so consideration and care must be taken.

1.5 Many drugs are based on food items, e.g. avocado for cardiac drugs, fish for betadine/iodine. Many drug 'shells' have lactose casings, so patients with an intolerance to lactose can't tolerate these medications.

1.6 Vicarious liability relates to the principle by which a practitioner's employer will take liability for the actions and omissions of the employee as long as they are acting within their job description and the boundaries approved by the employer.

Chapter 1 Test Your Knowledge

1　Immediately
2　When required or 'as required'
3　Prescribing, dispensing/preparation, administration, monitoring
4　Inhalation
5

　　(a)　90 kg × 20 mg = 1800 mg/h

　　(b)　$\dfrac{1800 \text{mg}/\text{h}}{1000 \text{mg}} \times 100 \text{mL} = 180 \text{mL}/\text{h}$

　　Note: did you remember to change the 1 g into 1000 mg to keep all the decimal units the same?

6　Right medicine, right dose, right route, right patient, right time
7　Over 230 million
8　Neonates (up to 1 month), Infants (up to 1 year), 1–6 years of age, 6–12 years of age
9　b-bockers
10　Absorption, Distribution, Metabolism, Excretion

CHAPTER 2

Activity 2.1

Pharmacokinetics deals with:

1　Absorption
2　Distribution
3　Metabolism
4　Excretion of drugs

Activity 2.2

Paracetamol has analgesic and antipyretic (fever-reducing) properties. It also has a morphine-sparing effect and can be used to reduce the total dose of an opioid. In other words, it increases the analgesic effect.

Activity 2.3

The pharmacist! Many hospitals have a drug information hotline that can be accessed via the telephone or computer. Better still, talk to them: they don't bite!

Chapter 2 Test Your Knowledge

1　Betty is more likely to be experiencing circulatory overload due to the infusion being delivered too rapidly. Inform the medic at once. This patient will require symptomatic relief by sitting up, close monitoring and oxygen. A fluid balance chart should have already have been commenced: keep these records accurate. Everything needs to be documented. In future, fluids should be administered through a pump and always checked regularly, especially if potassium has been added. This is a drug error.

2   No. This drug is contra-indicational in hypertension so she should not have been prescribed the medication. This is a prescription error.

3   Yes, as the prescription is all correct. The BNF states that the symptoms Daisy is experiencing are possible side effects. This is an adverse drug reaction.

4   Yes, this is a known side effect to the drug. Last time Michelle had this injection she had the same symptoms, but put them down to 'a night on the razzle' the previous evening. This is an adverse drug reaction.

5   Peter is showing signs of an allergic reaction. This is a medical emergency. Medics must be called immediately and the emergency drug box, containing adrenaline, etc., must be obtained and the adrenaline administered. When the emergency team have arrived the 'second-line' drugs can be prescribed and administered. The patient is having an anaphylaxis event, which is an medical emergency.

6   No, this is a drug error as the prescription is wrong. It should have been prescribed as 0.5–2 mg/kg two to three times a day, not to exceed 80 mg daily. The nurse who gave the drug as per the prescription chart is in the wrong, as well as the prescriber. This is a prescription error.

CHAPTER 3

Activity 3.1

Non-proprietary drug name	Proprietary drug name
Nitrazepam	Mogadon, Remnos
Sodium valproate	Orlept
Rivastigmine	Exelon
Pyrimethamine	Daraprim
Calcium salts/ calcium gluconate	Adcal, Cacit, Calcichew, Calcium-500, calcium-sandoz, Sandocal

Chapter 3 Questions

3.1 *Pro re nata* (when required)

3.2 AC means that the presence of food in the stomach may hinder absorption of a drug, which may then take longer to get into the system. CC means that there needs to be food in the stomach to protect the stomach lining, or the drug could possibly cause a stomach bleed. Do not chew: some drugs are enteric coated to protect the stomach lining or are long-acting/substained-release tablets and capsules. If these drugs are chewed the coating will be broken and they will no longer be long-acting or have sustained release.

3.3 Depot: a long-lasting injection, such as with contraceptives, antipsychotic injections and vitamin B_{12} injections. Intra-articular: an injection received in the articular space between two joints.

3.4 There are risks to vaccines of exposure to extremes in temperature. Vaccines need to be kept within a specific range as per the manufacturer's instructions and licensing conditions. If the temperature has not remained within the cold-chain parameters then vaccine is no longer a licenced product and should not be used. In such cases vaccines may become damaged and inactive, and immunisation will render no or little benefit and could cause harm.

Chapter 3 Test Your Knowledge

1 Prescription-Only Medicine.
2 This is the chemical or generic name. It is what we prefer to see on a hospital prescription chart.
3 This is the brand name or trademarked name of a drug.
4 This is when drugs are required to be kept within a specific temperature range of 2–8 °C during storage and transfer, e.g. vaccines.
5 1968. Most of us were not even born then – I wish!
6 Solutions, syrups, suspensions, emulsions.
7

PO	by mouth
mg	milligram
IM	intramuscular
g	gramme
IV	intravenous
kg	kilogramme
SC	subcutaneous
l	litre
PR	rectally
ml	millilitre
NJ	nasojejunal
TOP	topically
PV	vaginally
SL	sublingual
NEB	by nebuliser
OD	once daily
BD	twice daily
TDS	three times a day
QDS	four times a day
OM	in the morning
ON	at night
NG	nasogastric
PEG	percutaneous endoscopic gastrostomy

8 Cyclizine, Ondansertron, Metoclopramide, Prochlorperazine, Levomepromazine
9 Diuretics
10 These medications are a group of drugs whose main action is to reduce gastric acid production.

CHAPTER 4

Activity 4.1

1 1½ tablets
2 3 tablets
3 ½ tablet
4 ½ tablet
5 ½ tablet
6 ½ tablet

Activity 4.2

1

Side effect	Action/information
Constipation	Consider having PRN laxatives prescribed
Nausea and vomiting	Consider having antiemetics prescribed
Drowsiness	Often dose-related and temporary; have medic review patient
Respiratory depression	Should not occur if titrated correctly; have medic review patient

2 Naloxone: specifically designed to counteract the effects of the life-threatening depression of the central nervous system.

3 $\dfrac{5mg}{10mg} \times 5mL = 2.5mL$

4 $\dfrac{5mg}{10mg} \times 5mL = 2.5mL$

5 $\dfrac{7.5mg}{10mg} \times 5mL = 3.5mL$

6 $\dfrac{12mg}{10mg} \times 5mL = 6mL$

Activity 4.3

$\dfrac{20mL}{24hours} = 0.83mL / hour$

Activity 4.4

1 $50mg/1ml = 8-1 = 7ml$

2 $10mg \times 3 = 3ml$; $3ml$ diamorphine $+ 1ml$

cyclizine $= 4ml$, so $4ml$ ($8-4$) of water is required.

3 $8ml$ syringe $= 48mm$:
$48/24 = 2mm/h$

Activity 4.5

$\dfrac{50mL}{1hour} \times \dfrac{60drops / mL}{60minutes} = \dfrac{50drops}{perminute}$

Activity 4.6

$\dfrac{500mL}{25dropsperminute} \times \dfrac{15drops / mL}{60minutes}$
$= 5hours$

Activity 4.7

$12kg \times 40mg / kg = 480mg / day$

$\dfrac{480mg / day}{4} = 120mg / dose$

Activity 4.8

$\dfrac{48mL}{16hours} = 3mL / hour$

Chapter 4 Test Your Knowledge

1 $\dfrac{15mg}{10mg} = 1\frac{1}{2}tablets$

2 $\dfrac{15mg}{10mg} \times 1mL = 1.5mL$

3 $\dfrac{350mL}{3hours} \times \dfrac{15drops / mL}{60minutes}$
$= 29.166 = 29dropsperminute.$

4 $1000-700 = 300ml$ left to infuse.

5 $\dfrac{300mL}{20dropsperminute} \times \dfrac{20drops / mL}{60minutes}$
$= 5hours$

6 40 mg × 90 kg = 3600 mg per daily dose

7 $\dfrac{48\text{mL}}{12\text{hours}} = 4\text{mL / hour}$

CHAPTER 5

Activity 5.1

1 First, always ask the service user why, as you may be able to allay any fears. Then inform your line manager. Document. Never force someone to take their medication, i.e. using force. Question mental capacity. Speak to a pharmacist to see if a drug comes in any other form if the service user finds it hard to swallow.

2 Hold bottle and spoon/measuring cup at eye level to obtain accurate measurement. Check expiry date on bottle and when bottle was opened (shelf life). Check to see if instructions state that bottle must be shaken. Check storage instructions (should bottle be stored in fridge or at room temperature?). Close top as soon as possible (infection control).

3 Check with pharmacist; it may have an outer casing to protect the gullet. Never hide medications in food or drink. Check with pharmacist/GP whether medication comes in different format.

4 Wrong storage may destroy any active ingredients in medication. Brown bottles are used so that active ingredients are not destroyed by daylight/sunlight.

5 Medication has been sorted by pharmacist into boxes for each day's timed dosages; enough for one day, one week, or one month for ease of dispensing.

6 *Do not give.* Advise the service user of dangers of paracetamol overdose and the covert nature of paracetamol in over-the-counter medication, e.g. cough syrups, etc. Inform line manager, pharmacist and GP. Document why medication was not given.

Remember: all service users have the right to buy over-the-counter medication, the same as you and I (Deprivation of Liberty, the second part of the Mental Capacity Act).

7 Document, so that all medication tallies up with prescribed dosages, i.e. it does not look like you have given extra medication.

8 Some medications need to be given at set times to enable the drug to remain at controlled levels in the body (e.g. antibiotics, anti-epileptic drugs, etc.). Too-short gaps between drugs may be toxic. Too-long gaps between doses may mean the drug is not able to work to its optimal effect.

9 To mix contents of bottle well, such as the active ingredients in a syrup.

10 Inform GP/pharmacist. Think: should the service user go to hospital? Anaphylaxis?

Remember: it is always problematic when any new medication is given, as there may be a reaction. This often happens when a service user has been in hospital and medications are changed.

11 Same as expiry date. Do not exceed. Drug may become spoilt/inactive after this date.
Remember: once medication is opened, this will change.

12 Always use a 'no-touch' technique. May absorb active ingredients from drug onto your own hands. Think about infection control.

13 *Report and document.* Always admit your mistakes. The service user may require an antidote. A medic may give advice and instructions, e.g. to wash eyes with cool, boiled water, etc.

Chapter 5 Questions

5.1 Sublingual tablets are placed under the tongue. Buccal tablets are placed between the gum and cheek.

5.2 A mortar and pestle may cause cross-contamination. Specialist tablet crushers should be used.

Chapter 5 Test Your Knowledge

1 2 tablets, dose = 2000 mg per day

2 4 tablets; this is too many to give all at once. Ask the pharmacist to supply these tablets in a different format, such as 150 mg. Dose to be given in a glass of water, after food.

3 ½ capsule; these are capsules and cannot be halved. You will need to speak to the pharmacist again. The dose is 160 mg per day.

Activity 6.1

1 Rapid action is required. For example, patient is in severe pain and needs their analgesia as quickly as possible.

2 Drug is altered by intestinal secretions. For example, subcutaneous insulin.

3 Drug is not absorbed by the alimentary tract. For example, hydroxocobalamin (vitamin B_{12}) intramuscular injections.

4 Patient is unable to swallow: nil by mouth.

5 Drug is unavailable in oral form. For example, heparin.

Chapter 6 Question

6.1 Meniscus: 29.0 ml

Chapter 6 Test Your Knowledge

1 (i) Rapid action is required. Drug altered by intestinal secretions. (ii) Drug not absorbed by alimentary tract. (iii) Patient unable to swallow. (iv) Drug unavailable in oral form.

2 IM

3 SC

4 Not as mcg; it should be written out in full as 'micrograms' so as not to get confused with *milligrams*.

5 Yes. This is so the administrator does not absorb the medication through their own skin, and to minimise the amount of blood entering the body during needlestick accidents (as the gloves wipe off some of the blood from the needle).

6   Adenoviral vaccine

CHAPTER 7

Chapter 7 Test Your Knowledge

1   The procedure for administration is outlined in Table 7.1. However, this is a drug error because the BNF states that the correct prescription is 200 mg for three nights. Would you really have inserted four pessaries in one go? You will now need to document this as a drug error and inform the patient of your mistake, after talking to your line manager and a medic. Remember, you must always use your professional judgement and must not administer any drug just because it has been prescribed.

2   ADR is autonomic dysreflexia, which occurs in spinal patients only.
    Treatment plan
    - Sit the patient up (where possible) to induce an element of postural hypotension.
    - Ensure there is adequate urinary drainage (change the catheter if necessary, do not give a bladder washout/ instillation).

- Empty the rectum by digital removal of faeces (local anaesthetic gel should be used).
- Blood pressure should be treated until the cause is found and eliminated (administer a proprietary vasodilator, e.g. nifedipine, as prescribed).
- If unable to locate the cause, or symptoms persist, get help immediately.

CHAPTER 8

Chapter 8 Test Your Knowledge

1   The distance from the tip of an adult index finger to the first crease of that finger = 1 fingertip unit.
2   Approximately ½ fingertip unit
3   No, order a new tube. You need to go from the date the tube was opened and usually should discard it after three months, or less. Check with the pharmacist.
4   See procedure outlined in Table 8.5.

CHAPTER 9

Chapter 9 Question

9.1   PRN means *pro re nata*, or 'according to circumstances'. Commonly used to state 'as required'.

Chapter 9 Test Your Knowledge

Follow the steps given under the subsection Metered-Dose Inhaler in the chapter.

To clean the metered-dose inhaler the patient should wipe the mouthpiece after use with a dry or damp cloth or tissue. For aftercare, the patient will need to rinse their mouth out with water after the procedure.

CHAPTER 10

Activity 10.1

1 The drug is required quickly: the IV route is the fastest way to achieve a therapeutic effect from a drug.
2 Drugs administered by continuous infusion are given in order for adjustments to be made to the amounts administered; for example, insulin given via a pump to maintain blood glucose levels within tight parameters.
3 When a patient is unable to take oral medications; for example, when nil by mouth or unconscious.
4 When a patient is unable to adsorb medication orally; for example, patients with Crohn's or celiac disease.
5 When rapid correction of fluid or electrolytes is required; for example, patient has been haemorrhaging.
6 When other routes are not suitable; for example, a very young child with

reduced muscle mass is not able to tolerate IM injection.
7 When other routes are not acceptable to the patient; for example, IM injections may be refused by the patient.
8 When a drug is not be available in any other format; for example, glucose with sodium chloride.

Activity 10.2

Isotonic: 0.9% sodium chloride.
Hypotonic: 45% sodium chloride.
Hypertonic: 5% dextrose.

Activity 10.3

Oedema. Areas affected look puffy and when pressure is applied depressions or pits occur. Oedema may be localised due to injury or inflammation. Oedema may occur in the legs and ankles due to disease processes and can be relieved by elevating the legs.

Chapter 10 Question

10.1 Free flow can occur if the drip rate has not been worked out correctly, or the roller clamp not closed to the required position. The patient then receives an uncontrolled amount of the fluid or medication. In large amounts, fluid may overload the system, leading to over-infusion.
10.2 Speed shock is a systemic reaction that occurs when a substance that is foreign to the body is too rapidly introduced.

It occurs as a result of the speed with which medication is administered rather than the volume of drug/fluid. This can therefore occur even with small volumes. For example, furosemide can cause tinnitus/deafness if administered too quickly.

Chapter 10 Test Your Knowledge

1 Hypertonic
2 Every 72 hours
3 Every 12 hours
4 125 ml hour
5 $\dfrac{1000\text{mL}}{8\text{hours}} \times \dfrac{20\text{drops}/\text{mL}}{60\text{minutes}}$

   $= 41.66 = 42\text{drops per minute}$
6 $\dfrac{400\text{mL}}{3\text{hours}} \times \dfrac{15\text{drops}/\text{mL}}{60\text{minutes}}$

   $= 33.33 = 33\text{drops per min}$

CHAPTER 11

Activity 11.1

This drug should be given:

$\dfrac{\text{Dose}}{\text{Rate}} = \dfrac{20\text{mg}}{4\text{mg}/\text{minute}} = 5\text{minutes}$

Chapter 11 Test Your Knowledge

1 To make up to a total of 10 ml you need to add 8.5 ml of WFI. The solution is now 200 mg/ml.

2 Use the equation:
   Volume of drug to be given =
   $\dfrac{\text{what you want}}{\text{what you got}} \times \text{volume}$
   $\dfrac{1500\text{mg}}{2000\text{mg}} \times 10\text{mL} = 7.5\text{mL}$
3 7.35–7.45
4 pH 3.3–3.7

CHAPTER 12

Chapter 12 Test Your Knowledge

1
   (a) $\dfrac{20000\text{units}}{25000\text{units}} \times 1\text{mL} = 0.8\text{mL}$
   (b) Dilutant(48mL) – volume of drug$(0.8\text{mL}) = 47.2\text{mL}$
   (c) $\dfrac{48\text{mL}}{24\text{hours}} = 2\text{mL}/\text{hour}$

2 $3\,\text{ml} \times 3\,\text{hours} = 9.0\,\text{ml}$
   $3.5\,\text{ml} \times 2\,\text{hours} = 7.0\,\text{ml}$
   $2\,\text{ml} \times 2\,\text{hours} = 4.0\,\text{ml}$
   $2.5\,\text{ml} \times 1\,\text{hour} = 2.5\,\text{ml}$
   $4\,\text{ml} \times 1\,\text{hour} = 4.0\,\text{ml}$
   Total: 26.5 units of Actrapid have been received.

CHAPTER 13

Activity 13.1

If the end of the tube has gone down the bronchial tree tubes, instead of the oesophagus, the end will be in the lungs instead of the stomach or jejunum, causing serious harm or even death.

Chapter 13 Test Your Knowledge

The simple answer is to check with the pharmacist.

The propranolol is a modified-release medication so *should not* be put down the tube. This comes in a oral solution. The zopiclone is a tablet, so if the pharmacist agrees we may be able to crush it and put it down the tube.

Lactulose is a solution, and so it can go down the tube. However, check with the pharmacist first for drug interactions.

The fluoxetine comes in a capsule form so should not be split open and poured down the tube. A pharmacist should be asked to supply this medication in liquid form to be administered down the tube.

Actrapid insulin is to be given by subcutaneous injection; there is nothing to stop our patient receiving this injection. This drug has nothing to do with the nasogastric tube.

CHAPTER 14

1   Prescription charts, Oxygen monitors, NEWS 2 observation chart, Oxygen devices, staff training.
2   The safe positioning of patients onto their abdomens to aid breathing.
3   Breathlessness, agitation, confusion, tachycardia, tachypnoea, physical tiredness, increased work of breathing increased or decreased ventilation
4   24%

CHAPTER 15

Activity 15.1

M   Morphine
O   Oxygen
N   Nitrates (sublingual or IV), e.g. glyceryl trinitrate
A   Aspirin (300 mg STAT orally)

Chapter 15 Test Your Knowledge

1   Salicylates
2   Acetylcysteine
3   Monoamine oxidase inhibitor
4   Mature cheese, pickled herring, broad bean pods, meat- and yeast-extract spreads
5   Codeine phosphate, 8 mg; paracetamol, 500 mg
6   Adrenaline, amiodarone, lidocaine, atropine

CHAPTER 16

Activity 16.1

0   =   Awake and alert
1   =   Mild, occasionally drowsy but easy to rouse, or dozing intermittently
2   =   Moderate, often drowsy but easy to rouse, or responds to painful stimulus
3   =   Severe, difficult to rouse
S   =   Sleeping (some areas do not use this rating)

Activity 16.2

As we age, the following effects occur:

- slower absorption rate,
- slower metabolism rate,
- slow excretory time,
- opiates may be retained and be effective for longer periods, need to administer smaller doses (e.g. 1 mg IV in incremental doses) and extend the time between doses for an equal effect without complications.

Chapter 16 Test Your Knowledge

1 Acute pain
2 The WHO Analgesic Ladder shows these drugs to be effective in difficult-to-manage pain, in conjunction with analgesic medications.
3 Chronic neuropathic pain
4 The pain gate theory or Gate Control Theory: pulling out the hairs activates faster pain receptors to transmit the nociceptive stimulus to the dorsal horn of the spinal cord and 'blocks' the neuropathic pain signals, lessening the pain experience (it works for her!).
5 Adaption
6 A combination of the two therapies may work, such as analgesia and distraction.

Chapter 17 Case Studies Test Your Knowledge

17.1

Query	Answer
What is GI discomfort?	Gastrointestinal discomfort and includes stomach pain, heartburn, diarrhoea, constipation, nausea, vomitting
What does PO mean?	Latin for 'per os' meaning by mouth – orally
What does GTN – SL mean?	Glyceryl trinitrate sublingually – to be taken under the tongue
What is PV?	Administered per vagina
What is a daily INR test?	International Normalized Ratio test – used to check the blood clotting factor
What is a NSAID?	Non-steroidal anti-Inflammatory drug – used to control pain and inflammation
What does Nocte mean?	Latin for at night
What is a MR tablet?	Modified release – meaning tablet has coating that releases drug more slowly

ANSWERS TO ACTIVITIES AND QUESTIONS

Query	Answer
What does PR mean?	By rectum
What does 'monitor BG levels' mean?	Blood glucose testing
What does IDDM mean?	Insulin-Dependent Diabetes Mellitus – Type 1 diabetes
Why does a fluid chart need to be maintained for the patient prescribed Furosemide?	Furosemide significantly increases urination by inhibiting the reabsorption of sodium and chloride in the cells of the kidneys. This can lead to depletion of electrolytes if urine output +++
What does EC mean?	Enteric coated pill = polymer barrier that prevents its dissolution or disintegration in the stomach
What is a SL wafer?	Very thin sublingual drug
What does PC stand for?	Latin for post cibum = after meals
What does titrate to patients weight mean?	Finding the target dose of a medicine by weighing the patient and using the formula Weight (kg) X Dose so as not to overdose or underdose the patient

Query	Answer
What does QDS mean?	Latin for four times per day
What is a transdermal patch?	Like a plaster but impregnated with a drug so that when worn the drug is absorbed through the skin into the blood-stream
What is a FTU measurement?	Finger tip unit – a controlled measure of a drug in a cream
What does BD stand for?	Latin for Bis die = Twice a day
What does IM mean?	Intramuscular injection
What does OD stand for?	Once daily
Can you swallow the drug that states 'to chew'?	Always follow patient information leaflet/pharmacy instructions. If a drug such as Calcichew states that it should be sucked or chewed then this should be adhered to.

17.2 How many of these drugs (the top ten most prescribed generic drugs) have Stephen and Sarah seen on todays admissions to the unit? All of them.

17.3

Religion	Religious fact	Issues to consider	Answer
Buddhism	During the religious festival of Wesak, believers should 'refrain from taking substantial food after midday' (from noon to dawn).	A Client requires aspirin TDS, as prepared in his blister pack. How will this religious fact affect his medication administration?	Aspirin should be taken with food/after food (on a full stomach) – try to see if this medication can be taken in the morning with breakfast i.e. speak to Manager/GP.
Christianity	During the religious festival of Lent, many believers undertake observance of self-denial and commit to fasting or giving up certain luxuries as a form of penitence.	Could a medication administered to 'reduce pain' be considered as a luxury?	This depends on the service user – but try to persuade them that they need their medication but they can still give up another 'luxury'.
Hinduism	Most Hindus do not eat beef and/or pork and adhere to strict vegetarianism. The cow is the most revered animal for Hindus.	A client has been prescribed a capsule, which you have read in the Patient Information leaflet 'contains gelatine' – is this a problem/can the client still take this medication?	No – strict Hindus do not take any part of the sacred cow. Look in the BNF to see if the medication comes in a different format, i.e. tablet and speak to Manager/GP about the situation.

Religion	Religious fact	Issues to consider	Answer
Islam	Followers of Islam are called Muslims. During Ramadan, Muslims can eat and drink as long as the sun has set. Exempt from taking part in the Ramadan fast are: Children, the sick, the elderly, the mentally handicapped and anyone putting their health at serious risk by fasting, pregnant women and those on a tiring journey.	You notice that your client has 'cc' written on a bottle of medication sitting on the mantelpiece in their front room. Is this a problem for your Muslim client presently fasting?	CC is a Latin abbreviation meaning 'with food'. Try to persuade the service user that as they are classed as 'sick' they are exempt from fasting and they need to take food with their medication. At the end of the day, the service user with mental capacity can indeed refuse this advice. You will need to speak to your Manager and the service user's GP that the medication has not been taken, if this is the case and you will need to document this on the MARRS sheet.
Judaism	Passover is one of the most important festivals in the Jewish year. Four small glasses of wine are drunk during these celebrations in order to symbolise 'joy and happiness'.	Your client is taking a medication called Phenytoin for their epilepsy – do you have any concerns?	Many medications, such as Phenytoin, can not taken with alcohol. You will need to explain this to your client and document this in the MARRS. You should always discuss this with your manager and the Client's GP who may prescribe an alternative medication or change the times at least of the medication.

Religion	Religious fact	Issues to consider	Answer
Sikhism	Sikhism followers adhere to a system of Langar (or communal kitchen) – to demonstrate the need to share and have equally between all people.	Your client has popped out two of her prescribed cardiac pills from her blister pack to give to her sister, whom she states is experiencing 'flutters to her heart also'. Do you have any concerns about this?	Yes – individuals should **NEVER** swop medications. You will need to explain that you are aware of the principle of Langar, but the sister should visit her own GP to be prescribed the correct medication. This practice is extremely dangerous.

CHAPTER 18
KNOWLEDGE TEST

1. Prescribing, dispensing/ preparation, administration, monitoring (Chapter 1)
2. Right medicine, right dose, right route, right patient, right time (Chapter 1)
3. Injection and other non-oral routes (Chapter 2)
4. 100% bioavailability (Chapter 2)
5. The interaction of the drug within the body: what the *drug* does to the body. (Chapter 2)
6. The handling of a drug within the body: what the *body* does to the medicine. (Chapter 2)
7. When two or more drugs react with each other and cause unexpected side effects, or even increase the action of the drug. (Chapter 2)
8. Paracetamol (Chapter 2)
9. Harm caused by a drug at normal doses, during normal use. (Chapter 2)
10. The study of adverse drug reactions. (Chapter 2)
11. A yellow card (Chapter 2)
12. A patient information leaflet (Chapter 2)
13. General Sales List medicine (Chapter 3)
14. Prescription-Only Medicine (Chapter 3)
15. One to be taken three times a day (Chapter 3)
16. With food (Chapter 3)
17. A long-lasting injection (Chapter 3)
18. The need to keep medicines with the range of 2–8 °C at every step of the process: in storage (fridge) and transportation. Otherwise the medication (e.g. vaccines) will spoil. (Chapter 3)
19. Class A, Class B, Class C (Chapter 3)
20. The trade name or brand name of a medicine (Chapter 3)
21. Ventolin (Chapter 3)
22. British National Formulary (Chapter 3)

23 Under the tongue (Chapter 5)

24 These tablets/capsules are coated with a substance that enables them to pass through the stomach to the intestine unchanged. (Chapter 5)

25 (Chapter 5)

Drug	Possible side effects
Analgesics containing codeine	Constipation, abdominal pain, anorexia, seizures, malaise, hypothermia
Antidepressants, antiparkinsonian drugs	Dry mouth, vomiting, fatigue, psychoses, hallucinations, confusion, postural hypotension
Antibiotic allergy, non-steroidal anti-inflammatory drugs (NSAIDs)	Rashes, anaphylaxis, nausea, vomiting, diarrhoea
Blood-pressure medication	Unstable gait, fainting, light-headedness
Sleeping tablets, sedatives	Mental confusion, drowsiness

26 $225/150 = 1.5 = 1\frac{1}{2}$ tablets (Chapter 4)

27 $750/250 = 3$ tablets (Chapter 4)

28 $15/30 = 0.5 = \frac{1}{2}$ tablet (Chapter 4)

29 $150/300 = 0.5 = \frac{1}{2}$ tablet (Chapter 4)

30 $1g = 1000mg, \dfrac{1000mg}{500mg} \times 10mL$

$= 20mL (\text{Chapter } 4)$

31 $\dfrac{300microgams}{500micrograms} \times 2mL$

$= 1.2mL (\text{Chapter } 4)$

32 $\dfrac{750mg}{1000mg} \times 20mL = 15mL$

$(\text{Chapter } 4)$

33 Medication that is injected into muscle or the adipose tissue beneath the skin in order to be released gradually into the systemic circulation over a period of time. (Chapter 6)

34 The intramuscular (IM) injection route refers to injections into muscle. (Chapter 6)

35 The Z-track technique: pull the skin taut with the side of your non-dominant hand; the dominant hand inserts the needle; the dominant hand withdraws the plunger; after injecting, leave the needle in place for 10 seconds; keep the skin taut until after the needle is removed. The Z-track technique has been shown to result in less patient discomfort and fewer complications than the traditional IM method. (Chapter 6)

36 The subcutaneous (SC) injection route is in the subcutaneous tissue, meaning beneath the skin. (Chapter 6)

37 The intravenous (IV) route for injections is directly into a vein, via a cannula. (Chapter 10)

38 Intradermal means within the skin. The injection site used most commonly is the medial forearm area; it is mainly used for vaccines. (Chapter 6)

39 The cut-out part of the needle. (Chapter 6)

40 Not as mcg: it should be written out in full micrograms so it will not be confused with milligrams. (Chapter 5)

41 1.6 ml (Chapter 4)

42 1.2 ml (Chapter 4)

43 0.75 ml (Chapter 4)

44 2.4 ml (Chapter 4)

45 1.5 ml (Chapter 4)

46 0.6 ml (Chapter 4)

47 0.6 ml (Chapter 4)

48 14 ml/h (Chapter 4)

49 1.25 ml (Chapter 4)

50 5 ml per min (300 ml/h) (Chapter 4)

51 26 drops per minute (Chapter 4)

52 42 drops per minute (Chapter 4)

53 50 drops per minute (Chapter 4)

54 28 drops per minute (Chapter 4)

55 33 drops per minute (Chapter 4)

56 125 drops per minute (this is a 'thick' fluid and requires a blood giving set delivering 15 drops per ml). (Chapter 4)

57 The Bristol Stool Chart (Chapter 7)

58 Digital rectal examination. Remember that abbreviations *should not* be used in written care plans, medical records, etc., as mistakes can happen. (Chapter 7)

59 Atrial fibrillation (Chapter 1)

60 • Explain procedure to patient and gain consent.

   • Put on gloves and apron after washing your hands.

   • Check the following: right medicine is given, to the right patient, at the right time, in the right form, at the right dose.

   • Assist the patient into the appropriate position: supine with the knees drawn up and the legs parted.

   • Apply lubricating jelly to a swab and wipe the pessary. Some pessaries come with an applicator, into which the pessary is inserted.

   • Insert the pessary along the posterior vaginal wall and into the top of the vagina.

   • Wipe away any excess lubricating jelly from the patient's vulva with a swab or tissue.

   • Make the patient comfortable.

   • Remove gloves and apron (place in a clinical waste bag) and wash your hands.

   • Record the administration of the medication on the prescription chart. (Chapter 7)

61 One fingertip unit is the distance from the tip of an adult index finger to the first crease of that finger. (Chapter 8)

62 • Wash your hands.

   • Check the expiry date: write the date opened on the bottle and which ear Is to be treated (L or R).

   • Check that you are with the correct patient/service user. Check bottle for correct route. Gain consent.

   • Warm ear drops container in your hands (it may have been kept in the fridge). *Shake contents.*

- Position patient/service user. Draw liquid into dropper (if required).
- Check which ear is to have the drops.
- Administer drops. Replace top immediately. Leave head tilted for approximately five minutes.
- Wipe away excess.
- Use ear drops for full length of treatment.
- Avoid getting water in the ear while the patient/service user is having ear drops. (Chapter 8)

63 As required (Chapter 9)

64 Not shaking inhaler prior to use; floating the inhaler in water to determine whether medication is left in the device; not rinsing the mouth with water after administration. (Chapter 9)

65 It is an inhaler used every day to reduce inflammation in the lungs and slow down damage to the lungs over the long term. It should be used regularly, even if the individual user feels well. (Chapter 9)

66 By continuous infusion (Chapter 10)

67 This is a fluid that has the same osmolarity as plasma. (Chapter 10)

68 Hypertonic (Chapter 10)

69 135–145 mmol/l (Chapter 10)

70 Speed shock is a systemic reaction that occurs when a substance that is foreign to the body is introduced too rapidly. It occurs as a result of the speed with which medication is administered rather than the volume of drug/fluid. It can therefore occur even with small volumes, e.g. furosemide can cause tinnitus/deafness if administered too quickly. (Chapter 10)

71 This can occur if the drip rate has not been worked out correctly, or the roller clamp not closed to the required position. Patient then receives an uncontrolled amount of the fluid or medication. In large amounts, fluid may overload the system, leading to over infusion. (Chapter 10)

72 Achieve immediate effect; deliver high medicine levels; easier to prepare for practitioner than an infusion: no setting up of infusion devices; after administering the dose the practitioner does not need to monitor infusion devices as in continuous infusions. (Chapter 11)

73 Some drugs, especially antibiotics, have been freeze-dried. They are in solid form in the vial and need to be reconstituted with a known volume of solution before they can be administered. These powders can displace a certain amount of fluid, known as the displacement value of the drug, and this must be taken in to account when only part of the vial is being used. If this is not done, serious errors in dosage can occur and this is especially dangerous when working out paediatric doses, and those in critical care. (Chapter 11)

74 $5 - 0.2 = 4.8$ ml (Chapter 11)

75 Continuous intravenous infusion (Chapter 12)

76 May be used to maintain stable therapeutic concentrations of medicines, such as antibiotics. Infusion rate can be titrated according to a patient's needs, such as insulin to maintain set blood glucose levels. Allows medications with short elimination half-lives to be administered, such as adrenaline infusions in cardiac patients. Medications may be less irritating to the patient than bolus administrations. (Chapter 12)

77 Volume divided by time (Chapter 12)

78 26.5 units of Actrapid have been received. (Chapter 12)

79 Percutaneous endoscopic gastrostomy tube (Chapter 13)

80 Percutaneous endoscopic jejunostomy tube (Chapter 13)

81 Nasogastric tube (Chapter 13)

82 Continuous feeding via a pump; intermittent feeding via gravity; intermittent feeding via a pump; bolus feeding (Chapter 13)

83 Non-steroidal anti-inflammatory drugs (Chapter 14)

84 Gastro-intestinal irritation, increased bleeding time, bronchospasms in patients with asthma and skin reactions in hypersensitive individuals (Chapter 14)

85 Monoamine oxidase inhibitor (Chapter 14)

86 Mature cheese, pickled herring, broad bean pods, meat- and yeast-extract spreads.

87 Amiloride hydrochloride 2.5 mg, furosemide 20 mg (Chapter 14)

88 Amoxicillin 250 mg, clavulanic acid 125 mg (Chapter 14)

89 Aspirin to prevent blood clots; beta-blockers to help to protect the heart; ACE inhibitors to help protect the heart; statins to lower cholesterol levels. (Chapter 14)

90 $70 \text{ kg} \times 10 \text{ mg} = 700 \text{ mg/h}$ (Chapter 4)

91 $2.5 \text{ kg} \times 10 \text{ mg} = 25 \text{ mg}$ *daily*, divided by 3 (8-hourly) $= 8.3 \text{ mg}$ (Chapter 4)

92 $0.570 \text{ kg} \times 2 \text{ mg} = 1.14 \text{ mg}$ *daily* (Chapter 4)

93 120 mg/dose (Chapter 4)

94 900 mg/dose (Chapter 4)

95 540 mg/dose (Chapter 6)

96 Gentamicin indications - Septicaemia, Meningitis, Neonatal Sepsis

97 Ibuprofen indications - Mild to moderate pain. In children; post immunisation pyrexia

98 Gliclazide indications - Type 2 diabetes Mellitus

99 Dexamethason indications - Suppression inflammatory and allergic disorders, Croup, Cerebral, oedema, Vomiting with chemotherapy, Rhematic disease

100 Flupentixol indications - Schizophrenia and other psychoses

Appendix 1

SPECIFIC COMPETENCIES: MEDICINES MANAGEMENT

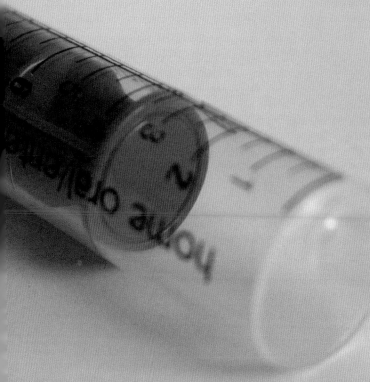

Medicine Management Skills for Nurses, Second Edition. Claire Boyd.
© 2022 John Wiley & Sons Ltd. Published 2022 by John Wiley & Sons Ltd.

KNOWLEDGE

	Performance criteria
1.1	The nurse/nursing associate can describe the therapeutic use of a range of medication to be administered.
1.2	The nurse/nursing associate can identify High Risk Drugs and critical medicines and has an awareness of the risks associated with use and timeliness of administration.
1.3	The nurse/nursing associate can state normal dosage of a selected range of medication to be administered.
1.4	The nurse/nursing associate can state the most common side effects of a selected range of medication to be administered.
1.5	The nurse/nursing associate can demonstrate competency in carrying out a range of physical observations linked to medication side effects.
1.6	The nurse/nursing associate has knowledge of poly-pharmacy risks and an awareness of monitoring and reporting systems.
1.7	The nurse/nursing associate can state the major cautions and contra-indications of each medicine to be administered.
1.8	The nurse/nursing associate can explain the intervention and actions to be taken in the event of a service user experiencing side effects.
1.9	The nurse/nursing associate can describe treatment strategies in relation to service user medication care plans. The nurse/nursing associate can explain the legal requirements relating to capacity to consent and the legal authority for treatment. The nurse/nursing associate can describe consent to treatment in relation to service user's detained in hospital under the Mental Health Act 1983. The nurse/nursing associate can describe the legal position in relation to consent to treatment for CTO patients; including community patients, patients recalled to hospital, and patients in hospital not recalled. The nurse/nursing associate can describe the legal position in relation to emergency treatment provisions where there is no authorising certificate.
1.10	The nurse/nursing associate can explain the importance of checking the prescription sheet, checking dosage, route/method of administration, validity or prescription, date and Doctor's signature.
1.11	The nurse/nursing associate can explain the importance of checking that the patient has no known allergies recorded on Prescription Sheet, and patients notes.

1.12	The nurse/nursing associate can explain the circumstances when telephone prescribing is acceptable and can describe the procedure as per the relevant PGN.
1.13	The nurse/nursing associate can explain the circumstances when prescribed medication would need to be omitted and can describe the reporting process for this.
1.14	The nurse/nursing associate can identify sources to obtain further information relating to medication – BNF, Pharmacist, Formulary, and relevant PGNs.
1.15	The nurse/nursing associate can describe the reporting procedure in the event of a medication incident/error as per hospital policy Web based incident reporting form.
1.16	The nurse/nursing associate can explain the process for supporting and observing service users in the event of a medication incident/error.
1.17	The nurse/nursing associate can explain the potential reasons and procedure for, and the implications of administering medication covertly as per PGN.

ADMINISTRATION

Performance criteria	
2.1	The nurse/nursing associate confirms the service user's identity/personal details; then checks for documented allergy status alerts.
2.2	The nurse/nursing associate checks the prescription sheet to ensure medications have not already been administered.
2.3	The nurse/nursing associate checks that the prescription is legible, valid, within BNF limits, signed, and dated by Doctor.
2.4	The nurse/nursing associate checks that authorisation and monitoring is in place for any medications that are prescribed above BNF limits or "off-label".
2.5	If applicable, the nurse/nursing associate checks the validity of Mental Health Act Forms against the prescription when medication is prescribed under the Mental Health Act.
2.6	The nurse/nursing associate checks the time of administration for each medication.
2.7	The nurse/nursing associate checks the route of administration of each medication.

(Continued)

	Performance criteria
2.8	The nurse/nursing associate ensures the correct administration of oral liquid medications using an appropriate oral/enteral syringe only.
2.9	The nurse/nursing associate identifies the name and strength of each medicine and selects the correct medication.
2.10	The nurse/nursing associate checks the dose of each medication and is able to calculate the correct dosage.
2.11	The nurse/nursing associate re-checks the dose and form of each medication and selects the correct one prior to dispensing.
2.12	The nurse/nursing associate measures the dosage correctly when administering all forms of medication including tablets and syrup.
	Enteral Routes. (If required; nurses/nursing associates who administer medication via enteral routes must be trained and competent).
2.13	The nurse/nursing associate will be aware of all routes of administration of medications and will develop competency as required; Buccal, Rectal, Enteral, Transdermal, etc., depending upon ward/patient need. If required nurses/nursing associates who administer medication via external routes must be trained and competent.
2.14	The nurse/nursing associate confirms the identity of the service user correctly before administering the medication.
2.15	The nurse/nursing associate makes a clear, accurate, and immediate record of all medication administered, intentionally withheld or refused by the service user; utilising the codes on the prescription sheet.
2.16	The nurse/nursing associate will gain consent as required and support service user rights to decline treatment and take actions as appropriate (reporting and documenting).
2.17	The nurse/nursing associate will not administer covert medication or administer medication in a unlicensed form (Crushed) without patient consent, MDT approval and plan in place, as per hospital policy.
2.18	The nurse/nursing associate demonstrates an awareness of the importance of completing the medication round with as little disruption as possible.
2.19	The nurse/nursing associate replenishes and checks stock levels and orders as required; using approved stationery and paper based or electronic systems. e.g. Automatic Drug Cupboards.
2.20	The nurse/nursing associate disposes of any medication appropriately.

HANDLING OF CONTROLLED DRUGS (FOR FIRST LEVEL REGISTERED NURSES). THIS SECTION DOES NOT APPLY TO NURSING ASSOCIATES

	Performance criteria
3.1	The nurse can define the schedules of CDs.
3.2	The nurse can demonstrate/describe the correct procedure for the ordering and transporting of CDs.
3.3	The nurse can demonstrate/describe the correct procedure for the receipt and storage of a Controlled Drug on a ward/unit.
3.4	The nurse can demonstrate/describe the correct procedure for the administration of Controlled Drugs.
3.5	The nurse can demonstrate the correct procedure for CD stock checks and management of discrepancies.
3.6	The nurse can explain the correct procedure for handling of CD cupboard keys, where appropriate.
3.7	The nurse can explain the correct procedure for the disposal of unwanted stock.
3.8	The nurse can explain the correct procedure for obtaining an emergency supply of CDs.
3.9	The nurse can explain the legal classification issues in relation to; CDs e.g. temazepam, phenobarbitone, benzodiazepines, tramadol, gabapentin, pregabalin.

RAPID TRANQUILLISATION (FOR FIRST LEVEL REGISTERED NURSES) – THIS SECTION DOES NOT APPLY TO NURSING ASSOCIATES

	Performance criteria
4.1	The nurse can define RT and has an understanding of the Pharmacological management pathway as per Trust policy.
4.2	The nurse can identify the medications used in RT and the routes/sites of administration
4.3	The nurse can state the aims of RT and when it would be appropriate to utilise RT

(Continued)

	Performance criteria
4.4	The nurse can describe alternative approaches to RT and can discuss the importance of staged interventions and de-escalation techniques.
4.5	The nurse can describe physical monitoring requirements around the use of RT and is competent in carrying out these observations
4.6	The nurse can explain the complications that can arise due to RT and describe when medical assistance would be required.
4.7	The nurse has an awareness of which service users would be identified as of a high risk with regard to the use of RT.
4.8	The nurse has an awareness of the need for post incident reviews and documentation after the use of RT.

Appendix 2
A TYPICAL PRESCRIPTION CHART

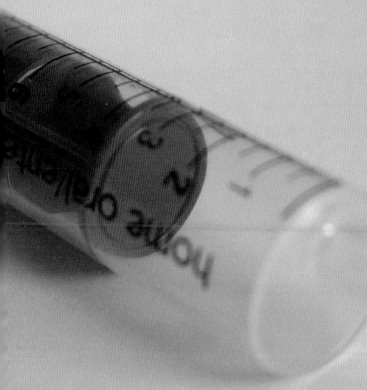

Medicine Management Skills for Nurses, Second Edition. Claire Boyd.
© 2022 John Wiley & Sons Ltd. Published 2022 by John Wiley & Sons Ltd.

North Bristol **NHS**
NHS Trust
IN-PATIENT PRESCRIPTION CHART

- AFFIX PATIENT IDENTIFICATION LABEL - (if available)		
SURNAME (MR/MRS/MISS)	DATE OF BIRTH	UNIT NUMBER
FIRST NAMES	SEX	CONSULTANT
ADDRESS		

PATIENT'S WEIGHT	PATIENT'S HEIGHT	PATIENT'S SURFACE AREA
(kg)	(cm)	(m³)

ENTER KNOWN DRUG ALLERGIES/SENSITIVITIES and their manifestations

WARD

Approved Healthcare Professionals Signature   BLEEP

OR WRITE NIL KNOWN

N.B. Patient must have RED allergy band if known sensitive

HOSPITAL

INSTRUCTIONS: Always follow medicines Management Policy for use of medicines

P H A R M A C Y

DOCTOR
1. Write all prescriptions in **BLOCK CAPITALS** and use **APPROVED** drug names.
2. Dose - state **CLEARLY**, for liquids/injections, state in terms of strength and volume where possible, e.g. 250mg (10ml); 2mg in 1ml.
3. As required prescriptions -- state the **MAXIMUM FREQUENCY** the drug can be given.
4. For discontinued drugs -- please date, sign appropriate box and draw a line through the cancelled item.
5. For additional therapy (e.g. anticoagulants/insulin), write as regular prescription, e.g. Warfarin -- as per chart.
6. All unclear prescriptions **MUST** be re-written to avoid errors.
7. Any changes of dose/frequency/route **MUST** be re-written to avoid errors.
8. After 15 days, when chart is full -- enter all current prescriptions on a **NEW** chart and file old one in patient's notes.
9. **MAXIMUM DURATIONS OF ANTIBIOTIC TREATMENT MUST BE DEFINED.**

NURSE
1. Check ALL sections to avoid omissions -- **ALWAYS** record why a drug is omitted.
2. If prescription is unclear, seek clarification **BEFORE** giving the medicine.
3. Nurse in charge to state administration times using 24 hour clock for ward/clinical area.
4. For patients who are self medicating record SM on chart.

Oxygen prescription Signed/Bleep: Date:
Risk factors for respiratory failure
Conditions associated with increased risk of hypercapnic respiratory failure (Tick if applies and prescribe oxygen in range 88 - 92%). Tick *None* if no risk factors present.

None ☐	Chest wall deformity ☐	COPD ☐
Morbid obesity ☐	Neuromusc. disease ☐	
Other ☐	Specify: _____	

Target saturations
(Circle correct range)
(Use high flow oxygen in cardiac arrest)

| 94 - 98% (Age <70 yrs) | 92 - 98% (Age >70 yrs) | 88 - 92% (Risk factors present) |

Oxygen prescription is mandatory except in an emergency

ONCE ONLY AND PREMEDICATION DRUGS

Date	Time	Drug (approved name - BLOCK CAPITALS)	Dose	Route	Doctor's Signature	Time Given	Given By	Checked By	Pharmacy Use

905204 (LGO)

- RECOMMENDED TIMES OF ADMISTRATION OF ANTIBIOTICS -	
6 hourly	06.00 – 12.00 – 18.00 – 23.00
8 hourly	06.00 – 14.00 – 22.00
12 hourly	09.00 – 21.00

- AFFIX PATIENT IDENTIFICATION LABEL - (if available)		
SURNAME (MR/MRS/MISS)	DATE OF BIRTH	UNIT NUMBER
FIRST NAMES	SEX	CONSULTANT
ADDRESS		

REGULAR PRESCRIPTIONS

	Date	Drug (approved name - BLOCK CAPITALS)	Dose	Route	Times of Admission	Other Directions/ Duration	Doctor's Signature	Date D'cont'd Sig.	Pharmacy
1									
2									
3									
4									
5									
6									
7									
8									
9									
10									
11									
12									
13									
14									
15									
16									

AS REQUIRED PRESCRIPTIONS

	Date	Drug (approved name - BLOCK CAPITALS)	Dose	Route	Directions	Maximum Frequency	Doctor's Signature	Date D'cont'd Sig.	Pharmacy
1									
2									
3									
4									
5									
6									
7									
8									
9									
10									

NURSE IN CHARGE
Complete times to be given according to "Guidelines for administering drugs"

INITIAL APPROPRIATE BOX ON ADMINISTRATION
When drug is not given – enter appropriate code only: for omitted doses or further explanations, complete exceptions to prescribed orders overleaf.

FOR AS REQUIRED PRESCRIPTIONS
Sign box in sequence, enter time given, and state dose (if variable).

Omission of a dose must be indicated by writing the appropriate non-administration code in the drug chart's administration section. An AIMS form must be completed when doses are missed resulting in care being compromised.

1. Allergic Reaction
2. Patient fasting
3. Omitted for clinical reasons*

4. Patient refused
5. Patient unavailable
6. Drug unavailable

reason for omission must be documented on the reverse of the in-patient chart

N.B. Recording non-availability of a medicine as a reason for non-administration is only acceptable AFTER confirmation from a pharmacist. All details relating to such incidents must be recorded in the nursing notes including the name of the pharmacist contacted.

REGULAR PRESCRIPTIONS – ADMINISTRATION RECORD

		Date	Date	Date	Date	Date
1	Time					
	Initials					
2	Time					
	Initials					
3	Time					
	Initials					
4	Time					
	Initials					
5	Time					
	Initials					
6	Time					
	Initials					
7	Time					
	Initials					
8	Time					
	Initials					
9	Time					
	Initials					
10	Time					
	Initials					
11	Time					
	Initials					
12	Time					
	Initials					
13	Time					
	Initials					
14	Time					
	Initials					
15	Time					
	Initials					
16	Time					
	Initials					

AS REQUIRED PRESCRIPTIONS – ADMINISTRATION RECORD

		Date	Date	Date	Date	Date
1	Time					
	Initials					
2	Time					
	Initials					
3	Time					
	Initials					
4	Time					
	Initials					
5	Time					
	Initials					
6	Time					
	Initials					
7	Time					
	Initials					
8	Time					
	Initials					
9	Time					
	Initials					
10	Time					
	Initials					

A TYPICAL PRESCRIPTION CHART

EXCEPTIONS TO PRESCRIBED ORDERS · FOR NURSING USE ONLY

Date	Time	Drug (approved name) and Dose	Signature	Reason

SPECIALIST WOUND CARE MANAGEMENT

Date	Site of Wound	Preparation	Directions	Size of Dressing (if applicable)	Signature	Pharmacy

TREATMENT FOR PATIENTS TO TAKE HOME

1. Prescriptions for take home drugs should be sent to the Pharmacy early in the day.
2. A minimum of **TWENTY-EIGHT DAYS SUPPLY** will be dispensed instead of fourteen.
3. **FIVE DAYS SUPPLY** will be dispensed for **ANTIBIOTICS**, unless otherwise ordered.

Date	Drug (approved name)	Dose	Route	Directions	Doctor's Signature	Pharmacy

Source: Reproduced here with permission from North Bristol NHS Trust and University Hospitals Bristol NHS Foundation Trust.

Index

Medicine Management Skills for Nurses, Second Edition. Claire Boyd.
© 2022 John Wiley & Sons Ltd. Published 2022 by John Wiley & Sons Ltd.